Overcoming Contraction

# Napoleon's Bathtub

Expanding Consciousness

## Jane Odin

Infinity Press
Taos, New Mexico

Jane Odin
www.janeodin.com


Infinity Press
Taos, New Mexico


Copyright © 2011 Jane Odin
ISBN 978-0-9679845-0-6

# Disclaimer

The information and recommendations in this book are based on extensive research, training, and personal experience. The exercises and techniques have been practiced by hundreds of people without incident.

The author does not give medical advice or prescribe any form of treatment. Application of exercises, techniques, general information and recommendations described herein are undertaken at the individuals own risk.

All the recommendations and procedures herein contained are made without guarantee by the author. It is your responsibility to research the accuracy, completeness and reliability of all opinions and information.

The author and publisher disclaim all liability in connection with the use of the information presented herein.

# Thank You

I wish to thank my ETW students and the following friends for their love, generosity, wisdom and support beyond the call of duty. Nat Jones, Bert Andrews, Bobby Cole, Ron Argelander, Chase Todd, Pete Denison, Lynne & David Trew, Lynda Ferris, Ann Stachura and Julia Armstrong. You have supported my spirit, my heart and my destiny.

# Dedication

This book is dedicated to all animal caregivers – wherever you are, whatever you do – to protect and enrich the lives of domestic pets, livestock and wild creatures. Many blessings to you and all the dear ones in your loving care.

# Contents

## Appendix

## Bibliography

# Prologue

This book is for those in search of *relaxation-on-demand* and *techniques for expanding consciousness*. It's designed for

- raising the frequency of personal awareness
- feeling good without medical intervention
- connecting with the Field, the web of vibrating frequencies that radiates throughout all space and all particles in the universe
- persevering with insight and vision in chaotic times

It gives techniques for maintaining the internal environment necessary for awaking to our extraordinary potential as radiant beings, vibrating love and joy throughout the Field of eternal becoming. It is a guide for further research into the process of transformation. You will know when you are on the inner journey because the world will not look the same.

Napoleon's Bathtub integrates a wide range of disciplines, creating an easy approach to knowledge that might otherwise take a life time to research and assimilate. Many great books exist on the subjects of relaxation, breathing, meditation, yoga, preventive medicine and quantum consciousness. But each is a vast study, all of which is difficult to master in today's world of never-ending emergencies. This book discusses a range of integrative approaches accessible to all comers.

Readers knowledgeable in New Age maneuvers will find much to ponder; perhaps you will learn to breathe diaphragmatically instead of sucking air into the upper lungs – or, develop reliable techniques of relaxation that work in the most stressful of times. Skeptics at heart may find sufficient proof that telepathy and parallel universes are worth exploring.

If you are middle-aged and don't breath diaphragmatically this is the book for you. It may take much practice to move away from *fight or flight* breathing. Persevere. It is a major change that enhances all aspects of health and well being. Once you get it you will never go back to the old way of heaving and puffing.

One needs a reliable process to counteract uptight configurations and reset normal. For example, when contraction becomes uncomfortable, take a hot tub and focus on the release discussed in "Don't Be a Tightass." Turn up the heat and dislodge the tightness moving upward toward the chest. Like Napoleon, I couldn't live without a tub; showers don't do the job.

There are many techniques for maintaining the flow of energy throughout the body including *stepping onto bending knees* when walking. This is difficult for some to achieve; instead they thud along on pogo sticks, moments away from a potential accident. The athlete, soldier and martial artist rarely move on locked knees. Solutions for maintaining bending knees are found in" Posture is the Foundation" and "Avoiding Falls".

My discoveries began as an actress/singer in NYC. Performing multiple shows every night required being centered, balanced and relaxed in order not to become an imitation of myself. I needed command of the relaxation process which was achieved by creating a network of checks, releases and balances activated with the ease of flicking a switch. This network is simply laid out – chapter by chapter.

Practice is necessary to experience the process and more practice is called for to maintain it. It's been awhile since I've had a client that practices. I need a magic wand, and damn those bad elves – they made off with it long ago. I advise staying with a practice until you know the experience as outlined in the *techniques/exercises* section. Be careful to follow the directions.

Being present for one's life 24/7 involves maintaining awareness of one's internal environment and responding to it in an appropriate manner. For example – illness often comes at night. One awakens at 2am with a stuffy nose or a headache or a pain in the side. Get up and attend to it immediately with natural remedies, yoga, rollers, shiatsu, hot tub and other preventive techniques. Never give it the opportunity to take hold.

While teaching at New York University I was amazed by encounters with *seeing* the pure energy of students. Sensitivity to light and shadow became a guiding reliability in often unusual situations such as the morning I gazed across the vast studio at a student who had a shadow over her neck and lower face, visible from over 50 feet away. I'll never forget her response to my query as she opened her mouth to show me: "*No problem. It's just my herpes outbreak.*"The back of her throat was covered with large sores creating an absence of radiating light. It was no wonder I could see it from a distance.

Sensitivity to light and shadow comes from wide-focus viewing discussed later in "Seeing Beyond the Obvious." This is an important skill; Castaneda referred to it as *seeing*. It enables one to view the entire picture instead of selective viewing, often influenced by habit and fear. It allows for noticing the tiniest change in surroundings.

Experiments in public places can have interesting results such as the first time I experienced wide-focus, in a NYC subway, one of my favorite places for exotic viewing. Although it happened 40+ years ago, in a state of total exhaustion, I remember where and how I sat in the train as the visuals began to unfold.

Whatever the circumstances, one must practice. No excuses. Excuses are a way of life; a nasty habit that prevents living in the moment and taking responsibility for one's destiny. No excuses are acceptable and here's an example of this reality.

Following a long illness, a student returned to the martial arts class of the great Budo Kai Kan Chief Grandmaster Rico Guy. Rico told him he must keep up with the class and no preferential treatment. The student became quite ill during the initial run-about exercise and retired to the john. After a reasonable time Rico called him to get back into the run and refused to show him any mercy. By the end of the class he was noticeably improved. I never knew a martial arts Sifu or piano teacher that accepted excuses.

I recall first meeting Rico around 3am; I was watering plants on the fire-escape with water pouring onto the sidewalk below. In the distance I saw a man moving in a steady run; he stopped under the dripping water and looked up. We said hello and I asked what was strapped on his back, to which he replied, "It's a milk crate filled with bricks." I was impressed.

My love affair with martial arts began when a music student invited me to a Kata (prearranged form) exhibition. I went and found myself sitting in a high school auditorium in NYC surrounded by serious looking martial types. Suddenly a man jogged down the long aisle and made a simple leap onto a very high stage. It was truly awesome. I watched him do a Kata that blew my mind and I knew this was for me. I speak of Grandmaster George Crayton whose high level awards fill pages. I was honored to hang out with him for several years and learn many things. And I practiced!

Throughout my martial arts studies I observed the healing power of the *arts*. On occasions, students arrived with noticeable flu symptoms and a general malaise. They practiced hard for 3 hours and concluded the class with most of the symptoms alleviated. Serious martial artists are masters of personal transformation; it takes incredible intestinal fortitude to attain desired techniques. It is an awesome process.

Napoleon's bathtub was the emperor's source of general well-being and so the reason for including plastics, artificial fragrances, and microwave frequencies in the Appendix - because these things radically interfere with good health and well being.

The sweat-lodge deaths prompted inclusion of the essay on plastics. Folks should have known not to do a sweat-lodge covered with plastic tarps. Apparently all involved were unaware of the toxic-off-gassing potential of soft plastics, particularly under the influence of intense heat. All tarps have warnings regarding ingredients. Somebody – out of all those in attendance – should have been aware of the dangers.

Kinesiologic *muscle testing* gives techniques for testing the effects of artificial fragrances and other chemicals on the body. It offers a reliable way of determining if aches and pains are serious conditions needing medical attention or just passing discomforts. With unbelievable, sky-rocketing medical expenses it's a boon to have insight as to the nature and seriousness of one's discomfort. Over the course of 30 years it has never failed me.

Some microwave frequency is impossible to avoid such as that radiating from cell towers, HAARP (see appendix), weather control experiments, Tesla wars and Homeland Security technology. The World Health Organization has warned cell-phones may cause cancer. Wonder if these admonitions will have any impact on those who keep the MW antenna strapped to their ears or on the bedside table. *Zapping the Masses* offers a brief, comprehensive review of accumulative microwave frequency as a major threat to good health and mental stability

Of course **love is the answer** – love and gratitude – for our lives and the extreme beauty and wisdom surrounding every moment. Love allows truth to soar above scary, heart breaking chaos and despair. The *Napoleon's Bathtub* techniques create the internal space – the relaxed-strength – to live life as a lover, transforming shadows along the way. Contraction is the heart of shadows; shadows of fear, shadows of illness, shadows of depression, and shadows of anger. Transforming shadows into light – whatever the technique – is the lesson and action for our time.

The elderly have an advantage in pursuing the inward-path. With more available time, less distractions and fewer obligations one can go on the journey of a lifetime into the subconscious and down the path toward a higher frequency of understanding. Expect nothing. The process in itself will reactivate every moment.

The *inner journey* demands hours of solitude and silence. That's the way it is – as witnessed by masters throughout the ages. The ancient sages hunkered down in small, freezing caves in order to arrive at their destination which was: maintaining open contact with the Field of all that is or ever has been. Initially this is impossible to accomplish when surrounded by distractions..

Throughout, reference is made to scientific research and ancient mystical philosophies that convey experiences, descriptions and disciplines that increase personal awareness and suggest wondrous possibilities for expanding consciousness into love, understanding, harmony, insight, joy and psychic awareness..

Thoreau wrote in 1856, "I went to the woods because I wished to live deliberately, to front only the essential facts of life, and see if I could learn what it had to teach, and not, when I came to die, discover that I had not lived."

Never before has there been a greater need for hyper-awareness in order to determine the real from the false at all levels of society. According to Ezekiel 28, duplicity has hounded mankind since Lucifer sprang forth as the bright and shining angel. "Thou wast perfect in thy ways from the day thou wast created, until iniquity was found in thee...All that know thee among the people shall be astonished at thee: thou shall be a terror..."

Lucifer is beautiful, a bright and shining light, full of deception, reminding one that the bad-guy rarely dresses in black and announces true intention. It's up to us to see past the glitter and promises of one's dreams coming true. One way or the other – we allow or create our realities.

*Overcome contraction*
*Maintain the flow*
*Connect with the Field*
*Enjoy the show.*

# Introduction

The book is arranged in brief chapters, allowing the reader to concentrate on one concept at a time until the objective is understood and perhaps accomplished. The chapters are ordered to present techniques necessary to accomplish the focus of the individual chapter. Breathing exercises are in initial chapters because following chapters demand the ability to breathe diaphragmatically. Just as the *bathtub exercise* is the first chapter because it is the easiest method for total relaxation, called for throughout.

Part One, "Overcoming Contraction" is focused on experiencing the difference between expansion and contraction. When gripping tension occurs, one becomes aware and able to release the discomfort. The heart of this work is in the breath and demands mastering diaphragmatic breathing. Excellent posture and absolute relaxation allow the breath to flow with healing power. Shiatsu, posture, and meditation maintain a release from contraction and allow one to live in the moment and experience psychic vision. All one must do is practice.

Part Two: "Expanding Consciousness", concerns bimodal consciousness, preventive medicine, psychic awareness, techniques of frequency expansion and theories of consciousness as related to the Field, which is both origin and destiny of all energy in the universe. We go into the details of what it means to be light-creatures and suggest what happens to *soul-energy* at the time of death.

Poems at the head of each chapter are examples of bi-modal processing. The words, sense of humor and rhyming are left-brain (LB) dominant and the emotion and content are right-brain (RB). If put to music the melody would be RB and the rhythmic articulation would be LB. This is discussed in the chapter on Bimodal Consciousness.

The appendix focuses on harmful frequencies in the environment. I've repeatedly heard folks say: "It's impossible to avoid nasties therefore I hardly give it a thought. It's a toxic world yet I don't see folks dropping dead around me." Wrong! They are dropping dead all around you – you're not seeing the connections – which pop out with careful research.

I've always followed a philosophy of *avoid as much poison as possible; it's bad for the health*. For example – years ago I was a smoker. My body could only take one poison so I cut out others such as fluoride, alcohol, negative relationships and nowhere work environments. I didn't live under heavy-load power lines and I've never had a cell phone. We'll peep into some of these arenas with several short essays on current environmental hazards.

Personal experiences and the experiences of students and clients are used throughout. For example, an eminent doctor from an outstanding NYC hospital once advised, "There's a tumor the size of a small grapefruit in your uterus. You must have a hysterectomy immediately." I replied, "I'll work on it for several months at which point we can check out what's happening." To his amazement, the tumor was gone in four months. That was very many years ago and it hasn't returned.

These are basic exercises and many readers will say – "Oh I know how to do this, I know all about it." This may not be so. Over and over folks claim to know all there is to know about the healing arts and they haven't a clue about basic diaphragmatic breathing. I was recently amazed when an experienced singer demonstrated proper breathing by lifting shoulders and heaving into the upper chest.

Diaphragmatic breathing is the core discipline without which little else will fall into place. Contrary to somewhat popular belief the lungs are not up high under the neck. Should anyone illustrate good breathing techniques by swelling the upper chest – don't waste your time.

"Connecting with the Field" looks at details of what it means to be composed of light and water in a universe of pulsing vibration. It considers relationships between the Field, expanded awareness and exceptional communication. Understanding these connections invites psychic intention to experience new realities.

Traditional religious beliefs in heaven vs. hell reinforce judgmental attitudes while misinforming daily reality. Knowledge of the Field suggests amazing possibilities for transformation. When you know the profile of biophotons, water molecules and communication in the quantum world you realize the potential for love, peace, hope, insight and wellness.

We recognize only what we are prepared in advance to see. Super-realities and hyper consciousness are missed when unaware of the possibilities. Knowledge of a subject invites that reality to live in one's heart and manifest as an ever-changing dance of truth and wonder.

# Part One

# Overcoming Contraction

*Jump in the water*
*Splash like a duck*
*Stay there a while &*
*Dream your good luck.*

# Napoleon's Bathtub

*"The only things which the Emperor finds indispensable are open fires and hot baths…Whenever he gets out of his carriage a hot bath is ready for him. If his nerves are utterly exhausted, he soothes them in a hot bath. When the war with England broke out he worked continuously, with four secretaries, for three days and three nights and then spent six hours in his bath dictating dispatches." Napoleon,* Emil Ludwig

Emperor Napoleon Bonaparte was an aggressive overachiever with an active imagination. He experienced radical mood changes, flipping between outbursts of temper and withdrawn depression; he probably had undiagnosed bipolar disorder. Hot-tubs were his method of coping and would have rated number one on his list of life's necessities. The tub was always in easy reach even on the battle grounds across Europe. He would sit in his tub, hidden behind bushes watching the battle rage on.

Heat and water are powerful therapy for anxiety, muscle aches, cancer and other systemic disease. Although we don't have the *luxury* of individual 41.8C water-circulating blankets used in cancer therapy, we have hot-tubs and saunas.

The New England Journal of Medicine reported the following regarding hot-tub therapy.

- Patients with Type 2 Diabetes Mellitus soaked for 30 minutes a day for 6 days a week. After 10 days they required reduced insulin, showed decreases in glycosylated hemoglobin & plasma glucose and improved sleep disorders.
- Participants experienced weight loss and cellulite reduction, losing a pound a week for 4 weeks.
- There was increased blood flow to skeletal muscles.

Native Americans use heat and water in ceremonial *sweat lodges*. Large rocks, heated in a blazing fire until glowing, are placed in a shallow, circular pit and participants sit close to the edge. Fiery rocks are added throughout the ceremony until maybe 70 glows in the pit. The number of rocks is determined by the purpose of the sweat which is always known before pit preparations begin.

A circular hood made of branches and covered with layers of blankets is placed over the ceremonial area before participants enter through a small flap opening. The lodge must be pitch-black, no light is allowed. Water is poured over the rocks and fiery steam fills the area. The heat and water intensify prayer energy and magnify healing from within. Water is poured over rocks throughout the ceremony.

Tiny infants and elders participate in sweats. The first one I attended was overwhelming; I thought my clothes were going to catch fire. When water is poured on the rocks, one is breathing fire. Many claim Native American sweat-lodge ceremonies heal life-threatening illness.

The 2010 James Ray sweat-lodge was unlike my experiences in Lakota sweats. Judging from photos and first-hand testaments it seems some participants in the Ray lodge were possibly sickened by off-gassing plastic tarps used to cover the sweats. I attended sweats weekly for years and never saw anyone made sick by the sweats. Plastic tarps were not used.

**Exercise**

Avoid dehydration by drinking a minimum of 8 ounces of water and no alcoholic beverages before the hot tub..

Light a candle and turn off the lights. Lie back so the water level is several inches above the neck. Sink totally into the experience.

As one enters the tub it's good to "pay respect to water, and feel love and gratitude, and receive vibrations with a positive attitude. Then water changes, you change, and I change. Because you and I are water." This quote from Masaru Emoto is found in *The True Power of Water* which describes water as the great memory holder.

After approximately five minutes, focus on breathing. Don't allow the shoulders and chest to rise toward the neck during inhalation. Think of breathing through the rectum; this image helps to initiate diaphragmatic breathing.

Release several long sighs and breathe slowly. Rest one hand at the waist and the other under the crotch. Direct the breath to expand the area under the hands and become one with the breath until the entire body is expanding outward from the midline of the body.

The aim is overcoming contraction. Regular hot tubs lessen the grip of tension before it takes control. Hot water neutralizes bad vibes, releases toxins, increases blood flow and unlocks gripped muscles. Heat and particularly hot water is one of the quickest ways of releasing pent-up anxiety and initiating slow diaphragmatic breathing.

When sitting at the computer for over three hours I often take a hot tub to stop the contraction process beginning to lift me out of the chair. Otherwise sensitivity to electromagnetic radiation will create a general malaise characterized by a slight nausea. Office workers might try splashing water on the face and whispering *love and gratitude* several times.

There are many well known, recognized hot tub therapies for muscle strain, arthritis and every kind of ache and pain. Saunas perform a similar function but are more severe than soaking in water. Water neutralizes negativity and always creates a soothing energy.

My dad set an excellent example throughout his lifetime. Every evening when he came in from working the range he went directly to the tub and turned on the hottest water and lay soaking for at least 30 minutes. He was in his 70's at the time and doing heavy labor on a large ranch.

Some folks refuse to take hot-tubs regularly. And when they do, they run a tiny bit of water into the tub and sit in the puddle for less than 5 minutes before getting out. Interestingly these folks are some of the most uptight, stress-filled people I know.

**Caution:** If you have high blood pressure or a heart problem don't use extremely hot water. Take a warm tub in a comfortable room. With experience you can determine length of time and degree of heat for the greatest relaxation. It's all right to feel a little light-headed. Splash cold water on your face from time to time or place a cool cloth on your forehead.

A very recent head injury is not compatible with hot tubs. The dilation of blood vessels causes the circulation of too much blood to the head. This could increase internal swelling which can cause death. My elderly mom died from soaking in hot water directly after a serious fall.

The elderly are advised to keep a container of drinking water close at hand and drink it throughout. A dehydration experience is very scary and comes with this caveat. If you should be in a standing position when dizziness occurs, lie down quickly on the floor to avoid fainting onto a hard surface. This is an extreme event that rarely occurs unless in a dry climate with inadequate hydration.

Recently a long time friend finally tried the hot tub approach to relaxation. He was a hard one to convince for whatever reason. From the first soaking he was transformed into a believer and now takes one every night. It has such a positive effect on him that he daydreams about it hours before hand. Not only does he relax but he has made it into a ritual with incense and candles which encourages mystical insights. May you have similar experiences.

*Don't suck it up*
*You'll create a draft.*
*Make life a joy;*
*Breathe through your ass.*

# Mastering the Breath

"Breathing is not merely an in-drawing and out-streaming of air, but a fundamental movement of a living whole, affecting the world of the body as well as the regions of soul and mind. From his breathing a man's whole attitude toward life can be read. Wrong breathing creates resistance to the fundamental rhythm of life and thereby makes self-becoming impossible." Karlfried Graf Von Durckheim

The power of diaphragmatic breathing is acknowledged throughout the world's religious philosophy, preventive medicine and martial arts. It reduces stress, improves health and transforms consciousness, producing greater effects on how one thinks and feels than food and exercise. Breath is spirit is life.

All creatures are born knowing how to breathe. Infants and toddlers display mid-torso expansion associated with diaphragmatic breathing. High chest breathing occurs by 7 years of age as part of developing self-consciousness and socialization.

Diaphragmatic breathing eases contraction around the heart muscle. Several days after open-heart surgery, breathing therapists retrain patients to breathe diaphragmatically. The process prevents tightening muscles from impeding blood flow and electricity through arteries and nervous system.

Descent of the diaphragm demands expansion in the mid-torso, promoting immediate release from contraction. Initially, it's difficult to expand and breathe diaphragmatically without basic relaxation techniques. The two processes work together. When diaphragmatic breathing becomes second nature, the uptight response no longer interferes with the breath.

**Benefits of Diaphragmatic Breathing:**

- Lung expansion occurs in the lower lung where oxygen exchange is most efficient.
- Aids in removing toxins from the lungs. The diaphragm pushes the abdominal organs down and forward which improves circulation and helps move gases out of the stomach and intestines.

- Radically lowers blood pressure in hypertension and brings relief from high anxiety states by lowering heart rate.
- Frees emotions strongly associated with pelvic region: fear, aggression, and sex.
- Releases upper body tension.
- Reduces stress hormones.
- Reduces lactic acid build-up in muscle tissue
- Produces inner calm and aids concentration.
- Supports the speaking voice preventing strain to vocal cords.
- Helps manage physical pain. This is one of the reasons it's central to La Maze natural birthing technique.

*Hara: The Vital Center of Man* was the only required reading for my classes at NYU. Every September Weiser Books would have over a hundred in stock ready for my students. It is a must read for anyone interested in the processes encouraged in this book. In it Durkheim refers to folks who have a high center as "push-overs." Carrying the weight of the body in the chest is a definite no-no for reasons of balance, power, control and grace. Diaphragmatic breathing moves the body-center into the pelvic region.

## Exercises

Exercises use three different positions: prone, seated and standing. In the learning stage it's easier to breathe diaphragmatically lying down and most difficult in a standing position.

- Lie on your back with knees touching and feet near the hips and hip width apart. This position pushes the lower-back to the floor and draws energy into the pelvis. Inhale through the nose to a slow 4 count. If this count is difficult do a 3 count inhale/6 count exhale or 2 count inhale/4 count exhale. The exhalation should always be through the mouth and twice the count of the inhalation.
- Place one hand on the upper chest and the other on the lower abdomen. Inhale and feel the lower abdomen expand. Don't allow the chest to move upward toward the neck. Keep the lower-back pushed down against the floor.
- Mentally extend physical boundaries and create a feeling of breathing into a being larger than yourself. **The abdominal area never becomes distended in a water-melon fashion.**

- Close your eyes and think of riding down through the body on the diaphragm *platform*. Or imagine a large disk dropping from the solar-plexus down to the pelvic floor as the inhalation is occurring. Objective of exercise is to breathe without lifting the chest and shoulders. It's easier to accomplish in a prone position.
- Lying down, inhale to a slow count of four. Direct focus toward the lower back. At the moment of inhalation, release muscles in the pelvic region, particularly the anal, sphincter muscles.
- Feel the pelvic region expand with the breath. Feel the upper and lower back spread and push against the floor with each inhalation. The upper torso, between the breast and neck, remains totally still. Exhale to a slow count of 8.
- Lie on stomach, arms to side, with shoulders touching the floor. Place backs of the hands against the mid-areas of each flank (gluteus maximus). Inhale, aiming the air toward the hands and feel the flanks expand outward in a horizontal direction.
- Blow out a vigorous, focused stream of air to a slow count of 10 (or less, if necessary). Imagine the breath moving down through the legs, out the feet and skin pores until no air is left in the body. Feel upward pressure against your hands throughout the exhalation. Repeat 10 times. High chest breathing will make it impossible to do 10 repetitions. If a problem arises, make sure you are practicing diaphragmatic breathing.
- Assume a low, squatting, frog position with the feet flat on the floor. If you can't balance, use a wall for back support. Blow out a vigorous stream of air. Feel a light pressure straight down from the coccyx (rectal area) toward the floor.
- Inhale, aiming breath for the coccyx. Feel the pelvic and lower back areas expand. Place fingers gently in the soft areas on both sides of the rectum and feel a strong pressure against the fingers. Look down and observe movement in legs and pelvis with each inhalation. Caution: Don't strain or push in the frog position as though constipated. The expansion occurs naturally with internal release.
- Stand with your back against a wall with lower back pressed flat against the wall. Legs are bent slightly. With hands on your waist, feel the back and sides expand with each breath. Move away from the wall and continue feeling expansion.

"A basic aim of diaphragmatic breathing is to stimulate directly the various organs in the body and to strain and relax the nervous system by modifying abdominal pressure through movement of diaphragm and abdominal muscles." Takashi Nakamura, *Oriental Breathing Therapy*

Zen Master Thich Nhat Hanh focuses on "mindful breathing" throughout his books and videos. He encourages the focus during all activities – while walking, sitting, working – because it is at the heart of personal transformation.

Mindful breathing means to be aware of inhalation and exhalation and nothing else. One thinks: I am inhaling, I am exhaling. Every breath brings one back to the *here and now* moment. It unifies body and mind, placing one in the present moment which is the first step toward greater awareness.

*Zen Breathing*, found in "Zen in the Martial Arts" tells a story of how breathing techniques saved the life of martial artist Joe Hyams when he became deadly ill with food poisoning. In the hospital, hooked to all sorts of devices he hears the MD inform his wife he may not survive. He writes, "I began forcing myself to regulate my breathing by taking deep belly-breaths (the stomach goes out during inhalation), holding for one, two, three seconds, and then forcefully expelling all the air. I repeated the process until I settled into a relaxed belly-breathing that required my concentration, inhaling through my nose for four counts and exhaling through my mouth for four breaths............Within a few minutes I was in control of myself and my body again." The MD's response at the time was "Incredible!"

You may have heard of Clif High, the computer programming genius who created a soft ware program that analyzes language patterns on the internet to make predictions about the future. When questioned regarding his excellent personal memory, he is known to have said, *once you can control your breath you can control anything in your body*. Indications are he speaks the truth.

*Release all the breath*
*Become an exhaler*
*Sing a sweet song*
*Let go of your failures.*

# Ride the Exhalation

"To his surprise and annoyance the beginner finds that mere knowledge of right breathing alone is of no avail. He knows what is required but cannot prevent the interference of the Ego. Again and again he resists exhalation halfway and assists the incoming breath. It's as if he dared not allow full exhalation. To accomplish this he has to learn above all to let go, to shift the point of gravity from above to below in his body and to achieve this he usually has to learn how to let the breath flow out fully." *Unknown*

Have you noticed the ease of extended inhalation and the difficulty of extended exhalation? Inhalation is automatic, exhalation requires internal release. The fear of *letting go* creates reluctant exhalers with habits of spasmodic breath-holding for up to 15 seconds. This is typical for stressed out folks. It's a control mechanism learned in early childhood. When the breath is held, thoughts and emotions are under control.

Lee Strasberg of Actor's Studio used the *song exercise* to initiate emotional response in blocked actors. The exercise was effective because once breath is flowing, emotions are released. Often actors would break into sobs midway through the song as they contacted unexpressed emotions.

Breath holding is visible from 100 feet away. I recall looking at NYU students from across an enormous warehouse-like studio and calling out to those holding their breaths. "How can you see from such a distance?" they asked. "Because it reduces the glow of light around the body" I responded.

Dr. Margaret Chesney at the National Institute of Health conducted research that found breath holding contributes to stress-related diseases by upsetting one's basic biochemistry: the kidneys reabsorb sodium, the body becomes acidic and the oxygen, carbon dioxide and nitric oxide levels are knocked out of balance.

This is bad news with regard to nitric oxide (NO) which plays a major role in transmitting messages between nerve-cells. NO plays a big role in many processes: memory, learning, inflammation, rheumatism, depression and the experience of pain.

You will notice there are no breathing exercises in this book that involve the *yoga breath count* which involves holding the breath for several beats between inhalation and exhalation. **Those exercises reinforce breath-holding tendencies which are at the root of many physical and mental problems.**

Breath-holding is a defense mechanism used to decrease outgoing and incoming stimuli and thereby control emotions. It also occurs when a physical task is a little beyond our ability. It's part of the grunt-push cycle and impractical for the following reasons:

- Aggravates stress
- Creates a general dullness and lack of awareness
- Produces contraction and retains incompatible energy that should be allowed to pass through the body.
- Interferes with communication.
- Causes the larynx to rise, which interferes with vocal production.
- Pushing and straining while holding the breath is known to produce heart-attacks. That's why so many folks die on the toilet.

As a professional singer, Chair of Voice Department (NYU) and private voice coach I know the problem of breath holding in voice production. It has a major tendency to cause the larynx to ride high thereby cutting off the flow of air. We speak and sing on the breath.

There are major connections between childhood emotional trauma, vocal strain, pitch problems and breath holding. Childhood trauma trains one to create breath holding patterns which greatly impact these arenas. Out of pitch singing is directly related to breath holding.

### Exercises

- Try speaking and holding the breath simultaneously. Listen to the sound of the voice. Now listen to the sound when you send out bursts of breath with spoken phrase. And finally, speak with a slow, steady stream of breath.
- Become obsessed with exhalation. Identify patterns of exhalation. Are you a chronic breath holder? What situations cause breath holding? Is breath holding accompanied by noticeable contraction such as tight rectal muscles or raised shoulders?
- Put a sign at home and work: Exhale! Exhale! Exhale! Try to catch yourself holding your breath and tell yourself throughout the day: *release, let go, exhale.*

- When tension and anger surface, release an extended exhalation. Blow breath out the mouth as slowly as possible. Try to extend the exhalation for 20 slow beats. Years ago I saw a Japanese Aikido master exhale for 200 slow beats. I counted them; it was awesome.
- Release ah sounds on long sustained breaths. Slowly increase the intensity of the sound until releasing a comfortable, sustained scream. Don't hold the breath when making sound. Should you feel uncomfortable in a seated or standing position, lie down and do the exercise. This goes for all breathing exercises.
- Focus on exhalation. Speak on the breath. A slow moving stream of breath flows from the mouth with each sentence. Hold your finger a few inches from your mouth and detect a very light stream of air as you speak. Now hold your breath and speak. Notice the difference in ease of delivery and quality of voice. The voice can be devoid of musical quality, power and even audibility when breath is held while speaking.

There's a tendency to hold breath when exercising. It's important to exhale with vigor at the difficult point of the exercise in order to avoid strain or injury. During intense physical action martial artists make sustained high-pitched sounds which indicate a strong release of air. Ride the exhalation.

*Blow away troubles*
*Blow away tears*
*Focus your breath*
*Conquer your fears.*

# Blow It Away

"Orientals believe that the breath is the first essential of life. They feel that only a sick man breathes with his upper chest." *Human Voice as a Weapon*, Timothy Hosey

John, a young actor experienced difficulty with breathing, audible speech and emotional expression. Frustration, anger and rage caused him to hold his breath, sometimes until his face turned red and blood vessels quivered in his neck. One time he fainted in class.

We tried several approaches and discovered blowing air with extreme vigor most helpful. Whenever he felt the anger coming on he released a long stream of air which enabled him to speak with a strong resonant voice. His first *blowing experience* outside the classroom was amusing and insightful.

Walking down a NYC street, John became angry when unable to avoid a childhood acquaintance who had crossed the street to corner him. In order to avoid fainting, John released a long, vigorous, focused exhalation. The acquaintance responded, "You can hit me, insult me, but don't blow on me" as he turned and walked away.

Animals are masters of *the blow*. They release loud blows through the nostrils when they sense danger. Equines flare nostrils and make a sound audible 1000+ feet away. My Chow made awesome blowing sounds when prowlers awakened her at night. It's an expression of intention and power.

The ultimate *blow* is the Kiai (spirit shout), a Japanese term used in martial arts, described as the release of all the breath in an explosion of sound. It involves the inner gathering of energy reputed to have the power to heal or kill, depending on how it is used.

Make sure your Kiai doesn't sound like a cry of fear. Make a spontaneous, low pitched, open vowel sound that comes from the Hara-Tanden (belly). The muscles in the abdomen become extremely tight in an outwardly direction. The Ki Society describes kiai as keeping "one point" in the Tanden. The sound must never come from the throat.

The kiai overcomes breath-holding and fear, making it useful with extreme activities. It's a method of channeling Ki energy. In Japan back in the old days it was translated as *meeting spirit* which generally means incorporating the weaker opponent into one's energy in order to control the person. Other translations define it as *spirit.*

Two NYU students, walking through Washington Square Park at night, became aware of 4 gang types trailing them. When thugs quickened pace, the couple turned, facing them and released a best version of the Kiai. The thugs took off running. A loud scream, releasing extreme air power, usually works to scare off attackers because they think you are crazed.

A Three Card Monte game/scam was set up directly in front of the entrance to my loft in NYC so that all comers had to pass through chaotic hostility. These were dangerous people who carried knives, threatened pedestrians and spoke no English. I appealed repeatedly to the police, got no help and finally had to deal with it myself.

I threw open the door, burst upon the sidewalk, kicked the cardboard boxes into the street and found myself surrounded by very angry Columbians who were screaming and gesturing wildly. I spontaneously worked the circle projecting every kind of air hiss one could ever imagine. I spoke the language of breath release and they were *blown away*, never to return and perch in front of 104 West 14 Street again.

This was a big moment in my personal growth. I realized, in the midst of the action, my knees were in an extremely low bend and my breath was coming from my Hara. I felt prepared to take them all on. I had no fear and it produced the desired effect. Blowing air is a technique worthy of mastering.

Holding the breath for any reason is not suggested. I'm aware it is a central component of the ancient and much revered Pranayama Yoga, which has many wondrous benefits for the advanced student. But for a majority, it may reinforce chronic breath-holding for emotional control. My experience has been that most folks need to practice a flowing diaphragmatic breath to avoid becoming less aware, less empathetic and less expressive. The first step will be to determine if you are a breath-holder by monitoring yourself throughout the day. If not, then Pranayama may be for you.

**Exercises**
- Blow a vigorous, focused stream of air through slightly puckered lips. Blow as though trying to put out a small fire. Do this 10 times in succession and repeat throughout the day.

- Once fairly proficient in the first chapters, practice sequential filling of the lungs by filling the lower lung first; the abdominal area will expand as the stomach and liver are pushed downward to allow the lower lungs to expand. The next expansion occurs at the waist area; 360 degree expansion occurs with waist and lower back expansion noticeable. The 3rd stage radically expands the back; it is felt strongest a few inches below the armpits. There must be no upward lift toward the neck and throat. Become proficient at this exercise to the point of inhaling and exhaling in three stages effortlessly. Try a series of 10 to build up diaphragmatic strength.
- This is an exercise for singers and greatly increases the power of the muscles involved in the exhalation process. Wear a tight belt round the waist; inhale and feel the waist expand against the belt. Hold onto the expansion as you exhale. Totally release all muscles at the end of the exhalation and do it again.
- Do a daily practice of blowing up balloons to increase lung capacity and strengthen diaphragm.
- Practice a hee-hee-ho-ho exercise releasing air on each sound for 3 cycles and then do an extended blow.
- Release a two syllable sound: wuh-ah. It's an expanding sound that is strongest in the middle of the sound as it moves from the wuh to the ah. Feel the body expand when releasing sound.
- When picking up heavy objects, opening stuck containers or executing difficult Yoga stretches release a steady stream of air. Never hold the breath while executing a task involving physical movement.
- Watch Bruce Lee's "Enter the Dragon" to hear beautiful Kiai.
- Practice releasing a silent, unnoticed stream of air when in an uptight social situation. Have the lips barely parted and make the release slow and consistent. Do the same immediately before going on stage to give a performance.
- Make a long series of single sounds releasing large bursts of air that explode from the body. Initially you will benefit from being in the Wing Chun stance (described in following chapter). It will draw energy into the lower body.

*Create a social revolution
Stop taking Viagra
It's not the solution.*

# Don't Be a Tightass

Wilhelm Reich's *Bioelectrical Investigation of Sexuality and Anxiety* finds tensing muscles of the pelvic floor makes sexual climax almost impossible for women. This should be of special interest to those who have never experienced the electrical charge at climax.

The pelvic floor is a group of large muscles creating a floor at the bottom of pelvis; the rectal canal transverses this floor. When the rectal muscles tighten, the spine is pushed upward, creating a feeling of internal pressure in the chest associated with stress. The upward push forces the larynx and glottis to lift and interferes with air flow. Releasing the rectal muscles creates a feeling of internal space. The pelvic floor drops and expands, allowing energy to flow into the lower half of the body. This release is essential for diaphragmatic breathing, relaxation and sexual climax.

Who coined the term *tightass* for uptight individuals? Did the discovery come from personal experience or observation? It's a great term, very descriptive of the process. The center of the pelvic floor, at the base of the spine is one of the first places to grip in the contraction cycle.

I recall standing on a subway platform observing two women, both wearing skin-tight pants, involved in a heated argument. Rectal muscles gripped in strained tension. As anger accelerated, sphincter muscles became tighter and tighter. During moments of reconciliation the muscles relaxed.

The pelvic floor is obviously the root of relaxation – as soon as the rectal muscles tighten – energy is on the rise to the chest and neck. Monitor the situation to determine if you have a problem and for the purpose of maintaining relaxation.

Breath is central to achieving release. Watch the front of the chest and you will see (and feel) the breath jumping up through the solar plexus. Place the outer edge of the hand between breasts and feel the breath rise. This is not desirable. Release the pelvic floor and initiate diaphragmatic breathing.

Men wishing to correct impotence without Viagra should focus on reversing tightass symptoms and improving diaphragmatic expansion. In some cases this remedy increases blood flow and energy transmission into the lower body which is just what is needed.

I recall practicing breathing exercises while walking the streets of NYC in the dead of bitter winter's nights. It was most difficult in older residential areas where there were no door ways to hide in, away from the wind. My objective would be to remain in a relaxed, expanded body - avoiding contraction and trembling from the cold. I slowed down the breath and maintained body expansion; soon I warmed up and unbuttoned my coat.

This was long before I knew the Wing Chun exercise, in which one stands with the feet at least 12 inches apart with the feet turned radically inward, then bend at the knees until the knees touch. Hold this position. Tuck the hips under slightly until the lower back is straight and the center of the head is directly in line with the tip of the spine. Stay in the position for at least 5 minutes. Breathe diaphragmatically with the knees always touching. The body may begin to tremble as the energy is forced into the hips and legs. Ignore the trembling. If you have a serious, undetected illness, the area of the problem will throb with an outstanding pain. This exercise will forcibly draw the energy into the lower part of the body and create a furnace that will melt ice.

During the exercise, if the pelvic floor is not released the body will tremble uncontrollably and the knees will not remain touching. Keep the lower back straight. Work with breath and discover your process for release. I used to hold the Wing Chun position for an hour every evening before Katas. Try it in a cold environment and find yourself slowly disrobing not unlike Tibetan monks in the dead of winter on the slopes of the Himalayas.

**Exercises**

- It helps to know if you're a chronic tightass. In a standing position tighten the rectal muscles super tight. Hold for a count of 5 and suddenly release the muscles. Do the tight/release several times until you're sensitive to the very different feelings. Can you feel the extreme expansion that occurs in the entire sacral-plex in particular the gluteus maximus at the moment of release? Stand for a few minutes with pelvic floor muscles relaxed. Do you feel the muscles trying to return to the tightass position? This indicates a chronic condition. We are creatures of habit and always want to return to what we're most familiar with. When the body experiences a more efficient and enjoyable way of doing something it quickly adjusts into that mode.

- Massage both flanks vigorously. Focus on pressure points located at the outer tips of the pelvic bone. The muscles should have a slight give when finger pressure is applied.
- Lie on your back with feet flat on the floor, knees pointing toward the sky. Make a fist with each hand and place them with the thumb-knuckle pointed up under the pressure points. Rock onto one fist at a time and rest all the body weight on the fist. Pressure is always applied at a 95 degree angle to the center of pressure point (or discomfort). Stay in this position until discomfort lessens, then rock onto the fist on the other side. Exercise can be performed on wooden rollers. If unavailable, use tennis balls, juggling balls or croquet balls. Place roller or ball under pressure point and rock hips until weight of body rests on top of the ball.
- Lean back on your hands in a seated position. Rock hips back and forth against the floor. Release pelvic floor muscles and pound one flank at a time against the floor. Hang loose.
- The American Physical Therapy Association finds a tight-ass creates tension in the lower back and recommends the following exercise to stretch the glutemus-maximus. Lie on the floor with the knees up and feet flat on floor. Put the ankle of the left leg on the right thigh and raise the legs toward the chest with the right hand. Do the stretch several times with each leg.
- A tightass interferes with diaphragmatic breathing. Try it! Create a tightass and try to breath diaphragmatically. It is almost impossible to accomplish.

*Create expansion
Relax in the groove
Contraction's a killer
And creates bad moods.*

# Overcoming Contraction

"You must confront and do battle with the two-headed dragon of fear and contraction. You need to understand how the fear and contraction of your power leads to your diminished capacity. You may not have the power to end your fear and contraction, but you will have seen it and you will have changed. From the expanded state you will have the power to see though the contraction, and that will give you real understanding. It will allow you to change the way you are living your life." *The Power to Create the Future*, Eric A. Mitchell

Once familiar with the expanded state, one becomes sensitive to moments of contraction as they occur. Contraction moves body energy inward and up toward the throat while creating a heavy, dense, out-of-balance and breathless feeling. Expansion feels light, airy, grounded, centered and flowing.

It's natural to pull inward, away from feared, offensive and unknown experiences. When this occurs contraction becomes the mode of generating energy. Notice the process as fear or anxiety take control. Breath-holding occurs as nerve energy pushes upward. The shoulders rise as the upper chest contracts. Rapid swallowing begins as the *pop your cork* scenario continues.

Contraction tightens muscles around the organs, glands and nerve plexus located along the internal midline. Contracting muscles signal *stress alert*, calling for the adrenals, pancreas and other hormone releasing glands to run a balancing act to one's disadvantage.

A strong contracting grip in the solar plexus is a cue for the hypothalamus via the pituitary to produce increased quantities of cortisol which can impair and eventually shut down the immune system. This is critical in our time when most immune systems are under attack by over-immunization, electromagnetic smog, off-gassing plastics, GMOs, microwave frequency and hundreds of toxic chemicals. We want to give the immune system as much support as possible.

The heart of tension is contraction. Stress is unavoidable but muscles can be trained to expand instead of recoiling into knots. **Overcoming con-**

**traction allows relaxation to occur while moving through tense situations.** It also prevents contraction from grabbing hold of negative energy found in all disease.

A young student experienced anxiety attacks to the point of almost passing out while driving. He described an inability to breath, "as though all the air had been sucked out of the car." We decided to monitor his high blood pressure while practicing slow diaphragmatic breathing. He was amazed as it dropped into a normal range. Diaphragmatic breathing and laughter exercises gave him control over his anxiety attacks while driving.

We express unique symptoms of contraction such as carrying hands in a fist position, crossing arms in front of the solar plexus, crossing the legs at the ankles and in front of pelvic region. Breath holding becomes involved when trying to withhold strong emotions.

It is difficult to feel good and enjoy life in a state of gripping contraction. Chronic contraction creates a rock-hard armor; internal energy flow and psychic guidance is radically impeded. We all know how difficult it is to communicate with an uptight person and we've all been that uptight person.

Most have experienced the joy of singing in the shower. The hot water is streaming down and the voice is strong and resonant. Try singing with the same strength, confidence and ease when out of the shower.

If your sound is conflicted, it is probably due to a closed throat or breath holding. A closed throat is caused by a raised larynx, produced by high chest breathing creating a high center in the sternum area. This pushes up against the vocal box, lifting the glottis and closing the throat.

Try making long, very extended *ah* sounds. The *ah* sound necessitates the back of the tongue being down which means the larynx will be down and the throat will open. When the back of the tongue is up, the larynx is in a raised position pushing it upward. Maintain the *ah* sound by listening to assure it doesn't become a uunh or uhhhh sound which occurs as the tongue lifts.

## Techniques

Lying on your back, envision a vertical line running through the center of the body from the center of the head, through the neck, torso and pelvic areas. Now tense the body all over. Start at the feet and move up the body making the legs, torso, arms and neck stiff as a board. Notice how muscles and bones pull inward toward the midline. Breathing becomes labored or ceases. Hold this position for ten slow beats before releasing. When releasing contraction be aware of muscles dropping away from the midline. There's a feeling of expansion and greater internal space.

- Close your eyes and *feel* the midline with the mind. Move up and down the midline until familiarity gives a sense of resting there. Repeat the exercise until you recognize the experience of contraction and expansion.
- Experience moment to moment emotions without allowing muscular contraction to occur. This is a good exercise to practice while watching scary movies or the evening news.
- Do a series of extended inhalations and exhalations. Feel the body expanding outward from the center line. Maintain the expansion while the exhalation occurs. It will immediately create an altered state of consciousness signified by an ear to ear smile.
- Contraction usually begins at the base of the spine and moves upward. It's almost impossible to be up-tight in one part of the body and relaxed elsewhere.
- Breathe! Expand! Release! Repeat the phrase mentally throughout the day. Feel the entire body expanding and releasing. It's difficult to be fearful, angry and uptight when *breathe, expand, release* is achieved in daily performance.
- Which muscles tighten immediately upon release? These muscles are habitually tight and need special attention. Breathe into the tightening areas. Feel the area expand with each breath. Visualize the muscles dropping away from contraction.
- When any unpleasant event begins to unfold, monitor muscles for contraction. Maintain diaphragmatic breathing as you check shoulders, neck, rectal muscles, toes and areas known to grip. Often the toes curl upward, back toward the body. It's an excellent sign the grip is on the move upward.

The following chapter will reinforce familiarity with the midline which is a focus for overcoming contraction.

*Try to feel the head and feet*
*The mind rests in the middle.*
*Feel them simultaneously*
*Float inside your breathing.*

# Consciousness Without an Object

Zen philosophy teaches understanding of self and aims to rid the mind of discursive thought, stop the habitual head-chatter and move toward the infinity of emptiness. A full container can receive no more. In becoming empty one perceives with an all-encompassing mind.

Two general categories of consciousness are inner directed without-an-object and outer directed with-an-object. Inner directed consciousness is the product of meditation, yoga and Tai Chi type activities. It enables introspective awareness and psychic vision.

Outer directed consciousness is goal oriented and concerned with achievement in the material world. It's the familiar consciousness of our time. Both modes have purpose when applied according to need. Problem is we're usually in consciousness-with-an-object.

Einstein moved between the two states of mind with great ease. He never worked with full concentration on a difficult problem for longer than 20 minutes. At which point he took a long walk, daydreamed as he enjoyed the country-side, confident a Eureka experience was in the making.

The following exercise is powerful. It creates a perfect state of mind for decision making, insight and feeling-good. The moment is experienced in fullest reality. Pain is moved outside the body, manifesting as an echo in the distance.

**Exercise**

Wear loose, comfortable clothing. Lie on your back, breathe slowly and gradually extend the exhalation to 8 beats. Move the mind down through the body from the head to the feet. Think of how your body feels in terms of density, temperature and general sensitivity.

Direct attention to the centre of the head and move through the body feeling the neck, shoulders, upper chest etc. Try to feel your feet. Concentrate on the feet until there's a sense of feeling them as totally as you feel any other part of the body.

Now, **try to feel the head and feet simultaneously.** The mind moves to the centre-line of the body where it is possible to feel ongoing contraction and expansion. This is the resting position for meditation, breathing, healing and intuitive awareness. You are at the heart of the matter.

One has the feeling of resting inside a bubble of energy while achieving greater objectivity. You feel the entire body receiving the inhalation – all the muscles move out from the centre-line, whereas contraction is experienced as a squeezing in on the centre-line.

Maintain focus. Keep returning to the intention of feeling both feet and head simultaneously. Over time you will recognize a distinct feeling of alert-spaciness. Take the intention into daily activities.

Rest on the centre-line when experiencing pain or fear. This focus moves one into wide-focus and creates sensitivity to the dynamic flow of energy. It automatically shifts perspective when accompanied by diaphragmatic breathing, giving one the sense of pain being outside the body.

Achievement isn't necessary to experience the benefits. The attempt to feel the head and feet simultaneously will automatically alter consciousness toward neutrality. Simultaneously focusing the mind in opposite directions causes immediate changes in perception as presented in "Inner Monologue" "Bimodal Consciousness", and "Techniques of Consciousness Expansion." It is the reconciliation of opposites, central to a higher level of consciousness.

When one maintains consciousness-*with*-an-object the focus is on marketplace mentality. One doesn't have to be a hoarder to generate consumer consciousness. Think about it; are you happiest when cruising the malls and looking for deals on the internet? Do you feel more alive after purchasing some new item? Is shopping a favorite pastime? The tendency is antagonistic to spiritual consciousness.

Living outside one's financial means is a good indication of rampant materialism which rarely morphs into a spirit based consciousness. The more one accumulates, the more is desired and the cycle of accumulation never ends. Apparently it's rewarding for some, but for one wishing to develop peace of mind and psychic awareness, it will be a difficult path.

As we face accelerating inflation under the control of evil bankers and deceptive, power crazy governments, we need greater control of tendencies toward extreme materialism. Try to go a month without spending a penny except for absolute necessities. Even if one is flush with money, try it as an exercise that will teach much, primarily because it is so hard to accomplish. We are programmed from birth to spend, spend, spend. It is an addiction greatly encouraged by government, ads, family and friends. Note how often one is urged to purchase something. It's really quite amazing.

Consciousness-with-an-object encourages one - do *this* and you will *receive that*. It makes many promises regarding feeling better because of purchasing power. Avoid the promise makers. Refuse to be a promise taker. There is usually a hidden agenda and the pleasure is often short lived as many learned in 2008.

**Consciousness without an object is the mode needed for the inward journey**. The final goal is a neutral bimodal consciousness with excursions into hemisphere dominance as discussed in Part 2. I'm certain many famous personalities – from Tina Turner to Thich Nhat Hanh and Leo Tolstoy – could tell us all about the process of maintaining the inward journey while creating meaningful balance and success in 3D reality.

Why mention Turner, Hanh and Tolstoy? They express the *integration of dichotomies* by living inner-directed and outer-directed lives simultaneously. Turner is a practicing Buddhist, indicating much meditation, *and* she is a magnificent singer/performer. Hanh is a meditating monk *and* a brave activist during the Vietnam War, saving boat people and leading non-violent civil disobedience. Tolstoy's encounter with Christianity transformed him from a self-absorbed aristocrat into the Father of social reform.

When the middle path becomes second nature - a place one can return to at will - connections referenced above are experienced firsthand. Overcoming extremism through the path of the middle-way produces radical change couched in radiant peace. It never encourages caste system mentality. There's no such thing as capitalistic democracy.

Undoubtedly many will find this perspective naïve and contrary to our way of life. Perhaps so, but this book is concerned with developing spirit based consciousness which can never condone the creation of a mass serfdom for the benefit of a greedy hierarchy.

*Don't look directly at it;*
*Look past it and you'll see*
*The truth is in the shadows of*
*The space between things.*

# Seeing Beyond the Obvious

"Our central nervous system is capable of being developed to such a point that we can tune in on any reality, from the very lowest mineral to the very highest spiritual levels…..The energy of a thought is broadcast in the form of electromagnetic waves and at the velocity of light into the environment and finally into the cosmos." *Stalking the Wild Pendulum*, Itzhak Bentov

How well do you *see* beyond the obvious. Are you aware of subtle change in the body? Does your psyche warn of impending danger? Are you sensitive to light emanating from all living entities? More often the active presence of unseen realities is revealed by the effect it has on us and the environment.

We live in a universe of twinkling light. All living things shimmer with a brilliance emanating from the flow of energy throughout the entity. Ability to see the ebb and flow of energy is possible. A first step toward *seeing* involves changing the focus of our camera-like eyes from narrow to wide focus.

Narrow-focus is used for left-brain viewing such as reading and detail analysis. It's the mode of academic pursuits. University graduates with advanced degrees are ingrained in narrow-focus, selective viewing. "Can't see the forest for the trees" applies to left-brain selective viewing, influenced by personal opinion and reflecting mirror images of the viewer.

Wide-focus is a right-brain technique, attuned to visual-spatial processing. As the visual mode of the creative process, it allows more light to enter the retina, making it the preferred mode for night vision. Wide-focus invites the entire picture to resonate as a whole. It's the way of *seeing* Don Juan teaches Castaneda in *Separate Realities*.

My first experience with wide-focus viewing occurred in a NYC subway. Mindless with exhaustion, I gazed, unfocused at the row of riders sitting across the aisle. Face muscles of the riders were moving slightly round the mouth area. It was apparent they were silently recalling detailed conversations. It was surreal.

I played around with wide-focus under different circumstances. Over time it became a reliable door to the invisible world. Layers of content, intention and purpose are revealed in simple communication with others. It's the *seeing* that allows one to experience auras radiating in a universe of shimmering light.

Nowadays I use wide-focus when walking in the forest and hope to see the shapes of light and shadow darting about. Often they are geometric shapes moving like birds through thick overgrowth. I haven't a clue what I'm seeing but it's delightful to experience.

Mode of viewing influences the bottom line of personal reality and determines the tendency of one's thinking process in terms of inductive or deductive reasoning. Wide-focus tends one toward deductive (whole to part) reasoning. Narrow-focus suggests reasoning from the part to the whole. The two rationalities create totally different perspectives. Ideally both are equally valid when used with understanding in appropriate situations.

It would be wonderful if Congress spent a day or two in wide focus. Actually it would be such a foreign experience for them, they would need extended workshops. Perhaps wide-focus viewing classes should be taught in high school.

Understanding the science behind wide-focus is relatively important in terms of convincing the uninitiated to use this mode more frequently. It gets a little complicated but here goes.

The periphery of the retina is composed of rods whose receptors are much more sensitive to light than cone dominated vision. It is the detection center and is always concentrated upon sensitivity at whatever sacrifice of form. **Rod vision is known as wide-focus seeing.**

In "The Hidden Order of Art", Anton Ehrenzweig defines rod-vision as necessary to reveal "the hidden order in the unconscious." He writes: "I will show that undifferentiated vision is altogether more acute in scanning complex structures. It treats all of them with equal impartiality, insignificant as they may look to normal vision. Normally our attention is drawn only to conspicuous features, the others sink back to form an insignificant ground. Wide-focus, syncretistic vision is impartial because it does not differentiate figure and ground." Lack of differentiation accommodates a wide range of incompatible forms. With attention dispersed over the entire visual field one is aware of countless relationships by which every element is connected, making it possible to detect the smallest degree of change. And since the rods are located at the periphery they really constitute "eyes in the back of our head".

Narrow-focus viewing relates to one thing at a time and the simultaneity of the moment is lost in the choice of the viewer to relate sequentially, "ordering" his vision to his particular taste. Learning and experience constitute most seeing, creating a manipulated view.

When wide-angle scanning is used in normal light, rods and cones are forced to function simultaneously. Focused vision alone is subjective and notices detail with accuracy whereas the detection of subtle change and subliminal qualities is more difficult. **Wide-focus is sensitive to the usually unseen whereas focus examines the already detected.**

Usually we scan from focused moment to focused moment. Our choices of focused examination are determined by need and expectation. Wide-focus brings an immediate change in experience. Sensitivity to energy is immediately increased; hidden relationships are revealed and the total experience is received.

Various cultures and people have practiced changing eye focus for survival such as the Moken natives known as the sea gypsies of Southeast Asia. Lynne McTaggart writes about their visual abilities in *The Bond* saying, "they have turned their eyes into cameras, changing the aperture at will." This is what we are talking about here.

According to ophthalmic biologist Anna Gislen, the Moken improve depth perception in order to effectively locate food on the bottom of the ocean. They constrict their pupils to a smaller diameter – just as a camera changes aperture. Without this ability to discern details, Moken would be diving for rocks and other non-food items.

McTaggart goes on to say it is the Moken ability *to see the space between things* that saved them from the tsunami. They noticed subtle changes in ocean tides, bird flight and swimming patterns of fish. With the environmental uncertainties rampant in our time – tornados, floods, forest fires, and earthquakes – we will benefit from practicing various apertures, using our eyes consciously in a camera like fashion.

We know from the work of Richard Nisbett, as presented in his '04 book *The Geography of Thought: How Asians and Westerners See Things Differently and Why*, that Chinese and Americans see things quite differently. Chinese view a photo with wide focus and see the entire picture equally while American's using narrow focus see only the central figure in the photo.

**Exercise**

Focus on a finger held 12 inches in front of your eyes. Maintain this focus and look around at surroundings. Is narrow-focus a familiar experience?

Now, close the eyes and focus on an imaginary object at a great distance. There's a feeling of looking into infinity. Open your eyes in wide-focus. Everything in your field-of- vision is equally seen.

There's a sense of looking past the thing viewed and yet taking in the entire object. There's no foreground and background. One becomes aware of the tiniest movement and shift of energy. Changes in the environment are noticed immediately.

Stare, in wide-focus, at several buildings (or any scene) at dusk. Keep each building equally in the gaze. Lights are on in windows, others are dark. You will see all objects equally. If a face comes to a window or a candle is lit in a room, even when at the edge of the viewing parameter, the change is detected immediately.

Try wide-focus viewing of various scenes and events. For example, a few friends, a room full of people or a full horizon of objects. You will see the subtlest change in attitude; true essence of personality; tone, shade and variations of energy flow. Practice makes perfect.

*The invisible world*
*Is just as real*
*As the favorite things*
*We see, touch and feel.*

# Electrochemical Creatures

We are broadcasting stations, sending and receiving according to personal attunements and environmental conditions. Thinking of oneself as a frequency processor encourages discovery of psychic possibilities and receptivity to the invisible world by way of regular contact with spiritual guidance from the Field (the space that exists between all things).

$E = MC\ 2$; *Mass is energy and energy has mass.* Einstein's Special Theory of Relativity presented a radically new vision of the world that transformed science, medicine, art, philosophy and metaphysics. I doubt many of the numerous movements occurring at the turn of the century such as Cubism, Futurism and Dada would have developed without Einstein's theory. Over a century later the news hasn't filtered down to the general public. Amazing! I sometimes ask "What do you think are the ramifications of our electrical nature?" Usually no one has a clue.

Mass (seeable material) and energy (wavelengths and frequencies) are synonymous and interchangeable. The invisible field is just as real as the material world we see, touch and feel. Objective physical reality is composed of oscillating electrical fields easily influenced by outside fields, whether natural (weather) or man-made. Living matter generates electric current and can be deeply affected by other frequencies such as microwave and ionizing radiation.

Microwave frequency is incompatible with human life. Many readers can recall the extreme warnings that originally accompanied microwave ovens. Now days microwave antennas are circulating throughout most homes and pulsing from gigantic cell towers. More on this found in "Zapping the Masses."

Psychoneuroimmuniology and Oriental medicine find negative emotions such as anxiety, fear and anger influence disease by altering flow and frequency of electro-chemistry. Effective stress reduction therapy is designed to maintain the flow of energy throughout the nervous system. This energy is known by many names such as qi, che, prana and the-force. Oriental medicine, Shiatsu, Acupuncture, Chinese martial arts, Reiki and Yoga sustain a general *intention* of maintaining the flow.

As Morpheus said in the Matrix"What is real? If you're talking about what you can feel, smell, taste and see, then real is simply electrical signals interpreted by the brain." Unfortunately we are unaware of electrical signals outside the visible range on the electromagnetic spectrum, unless under the influence of hallucinogens. This is why shaman and Indian cultures use the mushroom and other herbs to expand awareness into other realms.

Everything we take into the body affects electrochemistry, making diet a major focus in treating mental disease. Cells exchange mass and energy across membranes by processes under the influence of electrical potential; our chemistry is created & affected by electrical potential and vice versa.

So-called reality in the visible world is an illusion generated by the brain from electrochemical impulses. True reality is closer to a psychedelic state than to normal consciousness which is usually in the alpha or beta range.

**Alpha**: meditative state, healing frequency, appears in children at a round age 10

**Beta**: Concentration, learning experience, moderate stress, mild stimulants, agitation.

**Delta**: Depression, sedative drugs, alcohol, morphine, heroin

**Fast Beta**: Extreme anxiety, confusion, depersonalization, delusions of grandeur, extreme aggressiveness, cocaine (crack, crank) and other strong stimulants.

**Fast and Slow Wave Spindles**: meditation, desensitized pain, trance, clairvoyance

Look up electromagnetic spectrum on Wikipedia for an excellent overview of the various wavelength frequencies. You will find the classification of various radiations and their "main interactions with matter" most interesting. Several things catch my attention such as MW interactions termed "plasma oscillation" and "molecular rotation." Sounds like something we don't need.

You will notice we are in the middle of the EM spectrum, surrounded by frequencies known to be incompatible with our radiation and that includes MW frequency. There will come a time when it is recognized as the enemy of well-being.

"Birds of a feather flock together" and "You are known by the company you keep" are evident as undeniable truth. Have you ever seen creatures socialize outside their species unless thrown together under unusual circumstances? Could it be frequency based? Individuals of a species not only look alike, they share a common electromagnetic field attracting them to each other. They vibe the same frequency.

Rupert Sheldrake proposes that morphic fields are created by the repetition of behavior and other information establishing a morphic resonance which is a feedback frequency between the field and individual species. Although Sheldrake's theory continues to be a highly controversial notion it is similar to Jung's theory of the collective unconscious and the Vedic concept of the Akashic record, considered the record of all experiences and memories throughout all time. Morphic fields = Akashic record = the Field.

What does this mean in the real world? Look around at the folks you frequent. We are all one but apparently we are not all alike. No revelation, just an opportunity to learn more about who we are and with what we resonate.

My parents were generous with early childhood freedoms, although they recited the *birds of a feather* mantra from time to time. I could go bicycling, skating, hiking without being questioned as to details. But all social activities were carefully scrutinized and friends and acquaintances were introduced without fail. Now I understand why. They wanted to know who I was hanging with as evidence of where I was 'traveling' and the reality of my world.

**Exercises:**
- Meditate on the ramifications of our electrochemical natures. Look for evidence in routine places such as hospital instruments that read frequency and wavelength.
- Become aware of thoughts and feelings under the influence of changing weather, diet, people, music, entertainment, microwave frequency and natural environment.
- If you experience chronic physical discomfort such as nausea, keep a simple diary paralleling discomfort in certain environments and proximity to microwave frequency devices.
- Consider your social life and recall that likes attract. The placebo effect seems to support this idea.

*Doing the pogo walk*
*Thudding along in the dark*
*Wish I could bend my knees*
*And float with graceful ease.*

# Posture is the Foundation

"Many disorders of the body are frequently caused by interference with nerve transmission, due to the pressure, strain or tension placed upon the spinal cord, spinal nerve roots and surrounding tissue." *Chiropractic*, Arthur D.C. Scofield

The spine houses the nerve fibers connecting organs (heart, lungs, stomach, kidneys) and tissues to the central power supply. Millions of tiny fibers run through and twine around the spine. Bad posture distorts the natural curve of the spine, impinges on nerves and interferes with circulation in the nervous system.

Good posture creates internal space necessary to maintain diaphragmatic breathing. Zen and Hatha Yoga are taught in a lotus position which creates a straight lower back, allowing for easier transmission of nerve impulses and helping one recognize the ebb and flow of internal energy as part of moment to moment reality.

For decades posture was taught as an imperative for attractive appearance. The focus was on shoulders back, chest out and stomach sucked in. This advice is superficial and can interfere with basics of good health and physical grace.

Sucking in the stomach makes it impossible to breathe diaphragmatically. When shoulders are pulled back without corrected back-posture, shoulder and neck tension are experienced, often due to a sway-back.

Notice differences in the way people walk. Stick in the mud types walk pogo style on unbending knees. They have a noticeably uptight, graceless look. Athletes step onto bending knees. The head is centered directly over the rectum and the pelvis is vertical to the ground. The pelvic region is the strength of the body. Action originates in the pelvic center. When walking, the pelvis moves forward and the head and shoulders follow directly above the pelvis.

Poor posture can misshape a child's body for life. If there's an inherited scoliosis problem, posture is of even greater importance. A child's growing bones are malleable. Think of them as a growing tree. Practice good posture and the spine will be straighter than otherwise.

A talented 9 year old music student showed signs of early developing scoliosis and western medicine confirmed the diagnosis saying nothing could be done at the time. They advised waiting to see how it developed before acting. It was already interfering with her appearance and the way she walked so we immediately began work on the exercises included here.

It worked. Although we don't know what would have developed, we do know she quickly developed into a graceful dancer and lost the clumsy tendencies already developing. A young child's skeleton can be made straighter with exercise and positive thinking.

**Exercises**
- Study your posture in a full length mirror. Are both sides identical or is one shoulder and hip higher or lower than the other? Is the head tilted to left or right side? Walk toward the mirror from a distance. Watch for a balanced gait. Check out the side view. You may be surprised by what you see.
- Straighten the lower back by placing an imaginary board from the tip of the tail-bone to the mid-torso. Notice: **the knees must bend slightly in order to straighten the lower back.** The back can't remain straight with stiff, pogo-stick legs. As the knees straighten, the pelvis shifts backward to maintain balance while the head and neck shift forward. Looking in the mirror, bend the knees slightly and notice the sway-back disappear immediately. The shoulders fall into place with the head centered directly over the tail-bone. In this position it's impossible to slump shoulders, sway the back or carry the head out of alignment.
- Sway-backs are responsible for lower back, shoulder and neck discomfort. The weight of the body should rest in the pelvis not in the upper body.
- Sway backs are visually unattractive. Clothes can't hang as designed. The stomach sticks out and the buttocks protrude. The waist looks thicker from the front view because the hips are carried in a backward direction.
- Stand with lower back against the wall. Push the lower back toward the wall until the space behind the waist disappears. Become familiar with the feeling before stepping away from the wall. Never step onto straight knees or stand with locked knees.

- When seated keep the lower back straight from the tail bone up to the solar plexus. Don't allow the shoulders to slump forward and keep both feet flat on the floor. This will prevent many of the aches and pains associated with sitting at a computer all day. I sit at the computer in a lotus position because the position demands a straight lower back and keeps the energy flowing.
- Listen to the sound of your footfall when walking. Do the left and right sound identical? Or does one foot hit harder against the floor/ground than the other foot. If so it means the heavy hitting side is carrying a majority of the weight of the body. Check out the soles of your shoes to see if they are worn equally. Make necessary adjustment to create balance between the two sides.
- Imagine a rope attached to the center of the head pulling upward ever so slightly. Imagine another rope attached to the pelvis two inches below the navel and pulling forward as you walk. Although the head is pulled upward, have a strong sense of weighted feet echoing equally against the floor. You will be grounded and floating simultaneously.
- Hold the back erect in a seated position. A chair with a slight forward tilt will encourage an erect spine. Whatever the activity, don't slump into a curved spine. When reaching, bending, or moving in any direction keep the lower back straight from the tail-bone to the occipital ridge. Bending occurs where the legs insert into the torso.

*Maintain the flow*
*From head to toe.*
*Soon you'll know*
*How to fly.*

# Meridian Therapy

Channels of magnetic energy called meridians run up and down the entire body. Pressure points stimulated in Acupuncture, Shiatsu, and tapping are located along the meridian lines. The energy of the meridians, Chi or Ki, is the life force of the body and must be in a state of balance for health to be maintained.

The meridian system consists of:

*   12 main channels associated with the major organs they energize as revealed on an Autonomic Nervous System chart.
*   12 divergent channels that branch off the main channels as treated in *Shin So Shiatsu* by Tetsuro Saito.
*   Collateral channels that connect various pathways throughout the body.

It isn't necessary to know details of this complicated system in order to maintain energy flow throughout the channels. A general approach, using very basic Yoga, meridian stretching, Shiatsu, tapping and massage proves most helpful in removing blockage and balancing the flow.

Hatha Yoga is the formal system of meridian stretching. There are over 900 physical positions which clear blockage in the energy pathways and energize the internal organs associated with the meridians. Tapping, another method of stimulating and balancing the meridians, is possibly an easier, more immediate approach for those without the flexibility for Yoga or the knowledge of Shiatsu techniques.

I studied Shiatsu with Wataru Ohashi at the Shiatsu Education Center of America on West 55th in Manhattan. Looking back I recall the respect and love Ohashi generated toward students and patients. He also had a way of listening with his entire body. His soul resided in a meditative state.

One could see Shizuto Masanaga's (teacher) influence in the way Ohashi **always** moved, rooted in the Hara. This gentle, egoless man walked like a Samurai warrior. He was a living example of a major healing principal: all movement proceeds from the Hara. When one's energy rests in the upper body one is graceless and out of balance. You will find it interesting to shift into wide-focus and consider the movement-styles of those around you.

The following exercises generate energy through the meridian into the associated organ. They are also used for self-diagnosis. Stiffness and/or pain can indicate a problem. Initially, all meridians may be uncomfortable and inflexible. But when one or two meridians stand out as extremely painful, diagnostic muscle-testing is advisable for the purpose of initiating preventive measures.

Diaphragmatic breathing is a primary focus during Yoga meridian stretching, particularly for the novice and the elderly. Do the exercises slowly, releasing breath during the apex of the stretch. The release of breath will allow a deeper stretch and minimize possibility for injury. When the maximum stretch is reached, stay there for at least 5 slow breaths. Keep lower back straight by bending from below the hip where legs connect to pelvis.

**Exercises**

Yoga has a very wide range of asanas (positions); some are easier than others The following exercises are simple to execute and stimulate the associated organs by clearing the various meridians so energy can flow. That is what one is doing: moving energy and maintaining flexibility. The flowing energy maintains the integrity of the internal organs.

*Stomach and Spleen Meridians*: Kneel and sit back on your heels. Bend back until the upper body is flat on the floor. If it's too painful, use hands for support on both sides and ease back far as possible without tensing the rest of the body. This is an important concept: never tense the body when stretching. It negates the purpose of the exercise. Focus on the breath.

*Heart and Small Intestine Meridians*: In a seated position put bottoms of feet together and pull legs close to the body as possible. The knees are touching the floor. Hold the feet together with hands if necessary. Bend forward, bringing the arms and head to the floor in front of your feet. Stay there for several minutes and breathe slowly.

*Kidney and Bladder Meridians*: Stretch legs in front with feet side by side and touching. Bend forward from the pelvic area, keeping the lower back straight and lay head on knees. Stay in position until pain lessens.

*Liver and Gall Bladder*: In a seated position, spread your legs out as far as possible. Stretch out over each leg, lying down on each leg. Don't bounce when going down.

*Lung and Large Intestine*: In a standing position, straighten arms behind torso and grab hold of wrist. Bend forward and lift arms as high as possible.

The novice might start by simply bending forward and touching the toes, keeping the lower back and the legs straight. Stay in this position during the exhalation. Monitor your posture throughout the day, making sure you sit, bend, and reach with a straight lower back.

Stretching provides many benefits such as: increased circulation of blood & lymph throughout the body and increased flexibility. Practice tapping along the meridian lines that burn during the stretch. Tapping reinforces the stretch-release and helps unlock the flow of energy through the meridians.

Tapping has become a therapy called *Thought Field Therapy*, developed by Roger Callahan and considered quite effective by many practitioners. I first began tapping years ago when I had a ranch with large animals – donkeys, cows, mules and of course dogs and cats. I found tapping in the area of their occasional discomfort made them feel noticeably better.

Callahan's system uses primarily 10 points found on the head, chest and hand to release excess energy trapped in the meridians. I suggest tapping up and down stressed meridians to increase the flow. The internet has many videos and other information on the Callahan system. There is also a section on tapping in *The Living Matrix* (DVD).

## Callahan's Tapping Points

*Bladder* point is at the beginning of the eyebrows.

*Gall Bladder* point is at the sides of the eyes.

*Stomach* point is under the eyes on the upper ridge of the cheek bone.

*Governing Vessel* point is directly under the mid-nose.

*Conception Vessel* point is in the middle of the chin.

> (The Governing and Conception vessels are considered the main meridians of the bodies yin and yang energies. Tap these points daily.

*Kidney* points are an inch or so below the collar bone and in line with the centre of the eyes.

*Spleen* points are under the arm pits at the level of the breast nipple.

*Large Intestine* points are at the inside tip of the left index finger.

*Heart* point is on inside tip of the little finger. (This is an excellent point to stimulate with strong pressure on both sides of the finger. Do this by putting the finger between index and middle fingers of the right hand and squeeze.)

*Triple Warmer* point is on top of the left hand, in the grove directly below the knuckles between the little and ring finger. (Considered the thermo regulator, with the job of regulating bodily functions in the trunk. It is also associated with psychic channels and intuition.)

*Small Intestine* point is at the middle of the outside of left hand.

For those interested in learning more about Shiatsu meridians, purchase a wall version of Masunaga's Shiatsu Meridian Chart. You will find it an invaluable reference when stretching and tapping meridians. You might also wish to develop personal, yoga-based stretching exercises, using the chart as a general guide.

Deep penetrating Shiatsu along stiff, flaccid or painful meridians is powerful therapy which can be efficiently guided by Masunaga's Chart and book *Zen Shiatsu*. The bottom line is always how it works for you. If it doesn't provide relief from discomfort, it can be used as a diagnostic tool to pinpoint the problem before visiting an MD.

Yoga stretches all the meridians. But some of the asanas are quite difficult for older initiates; an excellent reason for children to get into the Yoga groove at an early age. It is excellent therapy for hyperactive and attention deficit children.

Practice basic Shiatsu on children and pets frequently. Combine with tapping over the chest and at the base of the neck. It's important to move fingers down the spine – one finger on either side of the spine, giving special attention to areas that push back at your fingers. Also try tapping down the center of the stomach area and also playful tapping over the stomach. Your child and pet will let you know how it's working.

Back in the day, as one drew closer to Actor's Studio on West 44th, NYC, Studio members identified themselves visually with self-shiatsu on the shoulders and neck as they walked down the sidewalk. From time to time one would run into members doing forms of self-massage on the subway and round-about town. Total relaxation was a primary focus at the Studio and many of Strasberg's exercises were focused in this arena. The purpose was expression of original personal behavior. It became known as The Method, as practiced by such film stars as Brando, Clift, Winters and Dean.

An example of the importance of relaxed muscles in Actor's Studio work in the 60's is found in the *sensory exercise* procedure. Several people would sit in chairs facing the audience and try to achieve a relaxed state. During the exercise Lee would creep about lifting arms to see if they immediately dropped back to their sides or remained where he placed it. He would always have a quizzical smile as he revealed the uptight participant whose arm remained frozen in space.

*Muscles read the frequency.*
*They will let you know*
*If you are with an illness*
*Or sick of the show.*

# Muscle Testing Diagnosis

Muscle testing is a diagnostic tool used in Applied Kinesiology; the muscles read the frequency of the area tested allowing areas of dysfunction to be diagnosed. After using muscle testing on clients for many years, I've never known it to fail. It has uncovered food allergies and diagnosed bleeding ulcers, Epstein Barr and an endless array of disease. It has also eased the minds of many who feared illness that didn't exist.

Imbalance in the body's energy fields such as the meridian system, can reveal problems before symptoms manifest. These imbalances can be read by muscle testing; it is a cornerstone of preventive medicine.

Meridian flow is affected by posture, mental stress and chemical imbalance. When extreme emotions or trauma are experienced, blood flow and electrical current are effected in such a way as to produce engrained reactions similar to past experiences in similar situations. And the process is reversible in that when an organ is irritated the associated meridian and muscles become imbalanced and memory-emotions can manifest as revealed in the following case.

A neighbor was experiencing chronic, severe stomach pain which was affecting his marriage. In this case he was subconsciously associating his problem with his wife's cooking. He had been to several MDs who were unable to diagnose the problem. He was scheduled to have a series of expensive food allergy tests when he came to see me. We muscle tested food he ate regularly and immediately discovered cheese was the culprit. He dropped the cheese and his problem ended.

## Technique

In order for the body to speak with clarity it helps to know the exact location of the internal organs, glands, nerve plexus, Shiatsu meridians and major muscle groups. Refer to an illustrated functional anatomy book when uncertain. Many folks don't have a clue as to where their colon, stomach, gall bladder, etc. reside. Please educate yourself.

Seated in a chair, hold the left-arm out to the side, shoulder height. The arm must be absolutely parallel to the floor. Have someone attempt to push the arm down with a gentle push. This isn't a battle of strength. The assistant applies just enough pressure to check that the arm holds its position. Don't overcompensate by raising your arm a tiny bit. Try to maintain the original position.

After left-arm strength is determined, put the right-hand directly over the area to be tested and hold the left-arm out to the side again. Have the assistant push down on the arm with a little less weight than known to move your arm down. If the arm drops under less pressure there is a problem in the area.

If you have digestive problems test the foods eaten regularly. Put a small amount of food in the mouth, chew it and hold it in the mouth while the left-arm is muscle tested. When the food is incompatible with your body, the arm will drop when tested.

Vitamins and medicine can be tested in the same way. After determining the vitamin is compatible, test the amount to be taken by piling a few on the chest. When your limit is reached, the arm will go flat.

An interesting test for smokers is to place an unlit cigarette in the mouth and watch the arm go flat. With the cigarette still in place, pile Vitamin C on the chest and the arm becomes stronger.

If you don't have an assistance to help with testing, you can use the Jug Method. Fill a gallon jug half full of water. If you're very strong, you may need more water. Stand or sit in a relaxed posture with the shoulders level. Hold the jug handle with the index finger of either hand, preferably the left. Keep the hand and wrist relaxed with the palm facing forward.

Slowly lift the jug until the arm is horizontal. Don't move or readjust the body while lifting the jug. If the jug is too heavy or too light, make the appropriate adjustment in jug contents. If the jug is a little too heavy to lift all the way with a straight arm, pour out a little of the contents and it will be the right weight.

Now you can muscle test whatever you want to test including food and chemicals such as Febreze. For example, hold a glass of milk in your right hand and lift the jug with your left arm. Or check out any internal area by placing your right hand over a specific organ and lift the jug.

It's possible to *surrogate test* infants, small children, the elderly and animals by placing your hand on the area to be tested and lifting the jug. With infants a Q-tip can be soaked with whatever needs to be tested and placed against the infants skin and the test will reveal allergies.

There is a rare condition that can prevent accuracy of the muscle test. When a person is seriously ill, a situation known as "switching" can occur and the person is referred to as "switched." This is when autonomic nervous system frequencies are skewed or reversed. Touch the tip of the pinky finger to the tip of the thumb and test the opposite arm. Test both sides and if one side tests negative there's a large probability you are switched. When both sides are switched it indicates an auto-immune problem.

MDs urge the patient not to self-diagnose but many of us can't afford to run to the doctor with every ache and pain? When we see an MD without having a clue to the problem, chance is, costly diagnostic tests will be called for to guide investigation. It's good to have some idea of where the problem exists before making a Doctor's appointment. Escalating medical expenses mandate the need for personal techniques to distinguish between disease and nervous tension.

Muscle testing is a reliable technique for self-diagnosis. There have been many times I thought I was dying only to determine it was stress related or a condition such as gas or muscle strain. I have found it to be a reliable diagnostic tool. The following exercise compliments muscle testing by offering additional information regarding general health.

Massage the entire surface of the body with the finger-pads, not the tips of the fingers. Exert an energetic pressure with the thumb in opposition to the four fingers. Focus on sensitive areas by applying pressure at a 95 degree angle directly into the sensitivity. Muscle-test areas that don't improve with massage. You might want to learn the meridian pathways, in terms of which physical organs they are associated with. This is helpful but not necessary to experience the benefits of the exercise. For further reference read Ohashi's *Do It Yourself Shiatsu* and Masunaga's *Zen Shiatsu*.

It's helpful to ask questions as to the general health of the body and the details of energy flow. The body has memory of all that has occurred throughout your life and will guide the search, suggesting areas in need of therapy and the techniques for relief.

*Roll it away*
*Roll it away*
*Don't allow discomfort to stay.*

# Roll Discomfort Away

Wooden rollers provide deep muscle acupressure synonymous with self maintained relaxation and pain relief. They're effective in relieving headache, backache, stiffness, intestinal discomfort and tension related pain. I've been using them since the '70s; my NYU students were known on campus by the rollers visible in their backpacks. The purpose here is to provide a guide for rolling discomfort away.

I recall traveling to India with the limited space of one backpack, in which was stuffed two wooden rollers - and I was sure happy to have them. I had a sciatica problem in my right hip and the roller was the only treatment that worked.

The roller is an excellent companion in Shiatsu sessions when the contraction has become locked. Although initially painful I can't recall a client that wasn't pleased with the results.

### Techniques

Never use a roller with aggressive, angular, hurried or careless movements. It's helpful to take a hot tub immediately preceding the roller session and from time to time repeat: breathe, release, expand.

Lie on your back and place the roller carefully so it doesn't touch the spine. Lift your hips off the floor and roll up and down the natural indentation on both sides of the spinal-column. Relax onto the roller. Feel the roller sink into the back. Don't allow the body to stiffen and push the roller out of position. Body weight must rest on the roller or it will jump around.

The first times you use the roller you may not be able to roll up and down the back. The discomfort could be too intense, so rest in one spot until the pain subsides and then move on to another area. Experiment in a gentle manner.

The delicate shifting of body weight allows the pressure to be aimed at a 90 degree angle to the problem area. After rolling up and down the back once, choose the area that hurts the most and stay there for awhile. Relax on the roller and you will feel the pain lessening.

Within 5 to 10 minutes, pain and discomfort will lessen dramatically. Often it will disappear. If the pain becomes more intense after 10 minutes, move on to another area and wait until a later session to return to the area of discomfort.

When familiar with the roller, purchase a second one to use in tandem with the first. For example, place R1 under the neck and R2 under the lower back. This relieves discomfort in the mid-back by pulling the energy in opposite directions, away from the problem.

Often I keep one roller at my neck while working other areas from the shoulders down to the lower back. In this position I feel little bursts of heat leaving my body as the contraction is released. It's important not to tense muscles. Slow breathing will maintain the release. If discomfort causes contraction and breath holding, the roller will not create the miraculous release it is known to accomplish. Let go, breath and sink into the roller – otherwise don't use it until you have a hot tub.

The roller stands in for fingers in unreachable areas on the back and pelvic girdle. For example, place a roller in the center of the gluteus maximus and hold in place with nearest hand. Rock onto the roller, lifting weight off the floor on the opposite side. Discomfort in the area indicates a tight bum needing release. This is central to stopping the tightass initiation of tension throughout the body.

**A shooting pain moving in a jagged fashion, radiating outward a distance from the roller, indicates the roller should not be used**. Try gentle stretching exercises, hot tubs, back brace, hard mattress or orthopedic pillow.

Unfortunately the rollers I used back in the day are no longer available. The Mini Back Roller is very similar but half the size. It can be found along with an array of other devices on Amazon.com. Some that caught my eye are: Body Back Buddy and Back Roller. You can also improvise with juggling balls and golf balls in a stocking, tied together with a knot in the middle.

Older readers can benefit from very simple maneuvers such as placing the roller at the occipital ridge, directly above the neck. Slowly turn the head from side to side, pressing against the roller as you turn. If it is extremely painful, massage the area with the three middle fingers (index, middle & ring).

The bedridden can place the roller on a hard book; it works beautifully to ease stress and initiate circulation throughout the body. Placed under the lower back it aids in moving painful gas out. For these reasons it's known to help hospital patients deal with the stagnation effect.

I have found the roller to be second only to hot water in relieving muscular tension and general contraction. In experienced hands it's a very powerful tool for deep muscle therapy. Check to determine you are not holding your breath, which is often the misguided effort to deal with discomfort.

If you are unable to find a roller, use the edge of tables, particularly coffee tables, to work on the neck. Lean back on the table edge from a chair or the floor. Initially you may want to use a towel across the edge to soften the touch. Slowly rotate the head back and forth, pausing on areas that are particularly sensitive. Allow need and imagination to guide efforts. For example, when hiking and camping I've been known to use the edge of a rock with a towel across the edge.

*Take a seat*
*Extend your light*
*Silence glows*
*Inside your mind.*

# Meditation Brings Truth

The Buddha was born to a royal family and lived in luxury until that fateful day when he left the confines of his family palace and discovered a world full of suffering and great misery. It was a horrifying experience for the young prince and he became determined to find a way to rid humanity of nightmare realities. His answer to *overcoming the suffering of mankind* is meditation.

Meditation doesn't lead to enlightenment, it is enlightenment - the two are synonymous and naturally create the transformation – that split second when one drops into the Field of total connection. Meditation is guaranteed to agitate the average, everyday, comfort zone by placing one in touch with insights that might otherwise go without recognition – which is a great blessing in times of baba sheepie and scary zeitgeists.

One is always encouraged to meditate without expectation but as Charles Tart writes in *Open Mind, Discriminating Mind* much always occurs when meditating. He shares a blow by blow description of the mindfulness meditation he practices which focuses on moment to moment physical sensations. It is an informative read detailing difficulties he experiences while meditating.

One finds a wide range of experiences in meditation, everything from greater awareness of internal processes to prophetic insight and inner peace. It is also a powerful way to impact the world and strengthen ones inner core.

On 3/11/2011 the world saw the Japanese people struggle to survive a devastating tsunami with self-control, kindness, consideration and great courage. Their behavior reflected centuries of meditation practice and generated a perfect model of behavior in times of great crisis. It was the antithesis of behavior seen in the Katrina storm in New Orleans.

Meditation has received much validation from the scientific community. Eileen Luders, a researcher in the Department of Neurology at UCLA discovered meditation changes the physical structure of the brain, creating more grey matter in areas concerned with regulating emotions, focus and mental flexibility. Regular meditation strengthens and creates connections between neurons. "These tiny changes, in thousands of connections, can lead to visible changes in the structure of the brain."

Antoine Lutz, scientist at Waisman Laboratory for Brain Imaging and Behavior at the University of Wisconsin, worked with Tibetan Buddhists with 20–40 years meditation experience and found higher amplitude and long-range global gamma synchrony which means an enhanced state of consciousness as their moment to moment reality. This remarkable study is reported in *Long-term meditators self-induce high-amplitude gamma synchrony during mental practice*, by Antoine Lutz, Lawrence Greischar, Nancy Rawlings, Mathieu Ricard and Richard Davidson.

If you have high blood pressure, try reading blood pressure before and after meditation. Regular meditation successfully lowers blood pressure and the more one meditates the more stabilized blood pressure becomes.

Studies report forty minutes of meditative visualization with diaphragmatic breathing increases the immune level response by creating significantly higher levels of IGA and Lysozyme.

There are endless types of meditation, giving one choice in finding a best practice. Some choices follow.

## Mindful Breathing
- Stay focused on the breath. Shallow, high-chest breathing is uncomfortable, prevents stillness and often causes rapid swallowing.
- The traditional Lotus position maintains a straight lower back. If necessary, sit in a straight back chair with both feet flat on the floor and the lower back pressed against the back of the chair.
- Breathe slowly and focus on long exhalations. Use the slowest breathing cycle maintainable without excessive effort. Perhaps a slow 2 count inhalation and 4 count exhalation is a good place to begin. Once breath and position are stabilized **don't move the body**.
- Focus totally on the breath; count the inhale and exhale. Do this while releasing the cycles of contraction moving up and down the spine. Remain with this focus for at least 20 minutes.

## Mantra
- Use a one word, one image or one sound Mantra. Clear the mind and focus on an external point such as a candle flame. Don't expect to receive anything from the meditation. Expectations destroy the

process. Guidance received is transmitted differently to each individual.

- Sometimes a clear image appears on the inner screen of the mind. Stay with the image. If it is a living entity (person, animal, tree) ask questions such as "Who are you? Why are you here? What is your wisdom?"
- A focal point is necessary to clear the clutter racing through the mind. After breathing is stabilized, experiment with various focal points such as a candle flame, mantra, or radiating light (discussed in part two.) When extraneous scripts (memory tapes) take over, return to initial focus on breath and resist temptations to adjust body and wiggle toes. Movement disconnects the internal process. Diaphragmatic breathing and total stillness are necessary for effective meditation.

## Inner Body

- Extend the *radiating light* practice by moving the light up the spine, connecting all the chakras, or focus on the midline until you feel the breath expanding out from this center line.
- Focus on a particular body organ by inhaling and exhaling into the center of focus and feel expansion in the area surrounding the organ. Send light and love to the afflicted area. From time to time repeat "love and gratitude."

## Reclining Meditation

In an effort to increase personal meditation time I discovered the pure joy of meditating in a reclining position. Judging from images of the Buddha, he did a lot of reclining meditation. It produces similar results as sitting meditation. The same techniques apply to make it work: total focus on diaphragmatic breathing and absolute stillness. This is an excellent approach for the elderly and sick. Make sure you do not cross the legs at the ankles.

## Tonglen

- This is a Tibetan Buddhist practice in which one inhales the suffering of others and exhales love, compassion, joy and success for all beings. The practice is known to reduce selfish attachment, develop compassion and expand loving kindness. It incorporates the *Six Perfections* of joyous effort, giving, ethics, wisdom, concentration and patience.

- Radiate light and focus on sending feelings of love and compassion out on the rays of light - to family, friends, relations and all beings, as you slowly exhale. On the inhalation embrace humility and selflessness while inhaling the deepest suffering for joyful transformation. Through the practice one becomes more empathetic, loving, understanding and compassionate.
- Focus on relieving the suffering of one person before moving to larger groups. Although one may not relieve suffering, one begins to cherish the importance of others. This is the Dali Lama's favorite meditation and one can see why, considering the great suffering of his people under Chinese rule.

According to multiple studies of compassionate meditation it reduces anxiety and inflammation while moving one into the place of compassionate love in the left frontal lobe. Negativity is found in the right prefrontal cortex; meditation and negativity do not have the same physiological origin or destination.

## Prayer

- Prayer is a practice similar to concentrative meditation; holding the focus is primary. The fewer words used the better. Lots of words bring distracting images that interfere with concentration.
- Cloistered monks were often instructed to repeat a phrase such as "Lord Jesus Christ, have mercy upon me!" 24/7 with the promise it would teach them everything.

Meditation gives one the ability to see as a child. It takes one past concern with the mundane and ordinary awareness. It should be a mandatory practice for children and adults alike. It would transform world consciousness. No doubt about it.

Ha-ha, ho-ho, hee-haw
200 times a day
Will keep the Doc away.
Join the laughing bankers.

# Laughter Heals

Writing in *Anatomy of an Illness,* Norman Cousins tells of healing ankylosing spondylitis, a rare, life-threatening disease with laughter. Chronic inflammation of the spine was fusing the vertebrae of his spine. Doctors gave him six months to live and sent him home to die.

With no other recourse, Cousins turned to laughter. He watched Chaplin, Marx Brothers, and Three-Stooges for hours every day. His illness turned around and 20 years later he was still alive.

Doctors should advise laughter to help cure disease. We know it works and it's certainly cheaper than bottled remedies and more fun to administer.

Why does laughter heal? Make sounds of laughter and note physical changes capable of transforming illness into health. The rectal muscles relax and expand; the entire pelvic region, mid-torso and back expand. Energy is generated throughout the body and the skin surface receives a gentle shaking in an outwardly direction. There's a strong feeling of total release.

Several interesting studies have been conducted regarding the effects of laughter on various aspects of health with the following results:

- Humor raises the level of infection fighting antibodies and increases immune cell count.
- Watching comedies lowered blood sugar levels in diabetic test subjects.

**Exercises**

- Express joy and laughter every day, particularly in hard times. The keyword is **express**. One may not be able to feel joy but the body and mind receive benefits from pretended experiences. Forced laughter is quickly transformed into the real thing. Pretending causes physiological change that produces the psychic mood of the action and the body responds accordingly.
- Make the sounds of laughter for at least 5 minutes in morning and evening. Pretense is fine. You'll find the pretense very quickly

turns into the real thing.

- The TV channel is easily turned from violence to comedy. Take charge of arenas where you can effect immediate change. If it makes you laugh it's good. Talk about what you love and avoid negativity.
- Chronically ill persons will benefit from a laughter project. Keep a record of the amount of time spend laughing each day. Create laughter several times throughout the day and determine the effect it has on both physical state and mental attitude. If laughter worked for Norman Cousins it should work for all of us.
- Rate the following arenas of expression from 0 - 10 according to joy and satisfaction received. If your score is low it is time to make some big changes. There's really no reason to slog along in the well worn rut of a mediocre life.

Hope for the future
Career
Mate
Spiritual development
Quality time with children
Quality time with friends
Positive emotional release
Financial security
Rest and relaxation
Artistic expression
Sexual gratification
Hobby or sport
Uplifting entertainment

Living in a state of limbo rarely transforms a situation for the good. Low scorers may be noticing recurring health problems i.e., flu, headaches, stomach problems, addictions. Over indulgence in food, alcohol and drugs are symptoms of the void.

A well known fable illustrates the power of pretense. A wise sage came upon a broken-hearted person sitting at the edge of a river. It was obvious he had been there for many months. The sage asked about his situation and the desolate one said "I have lost my home, my family and my reason for living." The sage replied, "Pretend to get up and walk down the road to visit neighbors. Then pretend to build a house and grow a garden.

Pretend to socialize everyday and the moment will come when pretense has magically turned into reality."

Return to our childhood laughter schedule – 300 times a day – whereas a 40 year old laughs 4 times a day and some folks don't laugh at all. Raise your daily laughter expression with phony laughter; the more fearful, depressed, anxious, enraged you are - the more laughter episodes are needed.

Laughter is such a simple, inexpensive solution – it would be a positive addition to all classrooms, hospital settings, jails and elderly centers. I would include CEO lounges but they already have ha-ha-rooms designated throughout their vast holdings. Hmmmm! There may be more to another old saying – *laughing all the way to the bank.*

Imagine laughter projects taking place in obviously appropriate places. It would cost nothing and be 100% effective. Several times a day, particularly in the morning and evening – everybody pretends to laugh for 5+ minutes. Not much to ask for the sake of improving health and general well being. It's a great idea to join all the laughing bankers.

*Present in the moment*
*Do not fear the night*
*Watch for bushy tails*
*Keep them well in sight.*

# Inner Monologue

Frame of mind is central to living a good life, mastering new skills, releasing creative expression and overcoming fear. A positive inner monologue allows intuition to guide one through all the little nooks and crannies in life.

The inner-monologue used for healing and achievement is one-voice, based in moment to moment action and devoid of negativity. Its expression is centered on action words - love, go, do, see, feel. Criticism is never allowed. Inner monologue moves toward a desired intention. Intention is the guiding focus that sets it apart from brain-hemisphere dialectics.

I recall an inner monologue experience that worked for me in a time of great stress. I was traveling by car from New Mexico to Rocky Mountain National Park. At the top of the Rockies I arrived at the Trail Ridge Road and froze in terror when I discovered the road in front of me was barely wide enough for two cars to squeeze past each other. There was maybe a foot of ground on the road-side and a sheer drop 1000's of feet down. There were no guard rails and the wind was howling around my high profile 4 Runner.

At first my inner monologue was devoid of intention and full of negativity. *No. No. This cannot be. This is insanity. I'll never make it. The road is too narrow, how can I get outta here?* This was quickly transformed into an appropriate monologue. *If that car can get across so can I. And since I'm up here I will look around at the view and see all there is to see of the mountains. Breathe slowly and enjoy the view.*

The following is an example of an inner monologue used to accomplish diaphragmatic breathing. *Breathe slowly, inhale 2, 3, 4, exhale 2, 3, 4, 5, 6, 7, 8. Release. Surrender. Let go of shoulders. Feel the upper back against the floor. Inhale 2, 3, 4, exhale 2, 3, 4, 5, 6, 7, 8. I am breathing 360 degrees out from the midline. I feel feet, head and hands simultaneously. Release pelvic floor and knees. Soft knees. I feel the breath expanding my legs and feet. I'm expanding, with each breath. The internal space is becoming larger and larger.*

**Technique**

The mind empties as focus centers in the breath. Imagine breathing through the skin pores, keeping in mind the following suggestions.

- Meditate upon intention. Compose a brief command and repeat it slowly to yourself. Stay focused.
- Intention rests in being focused on the meditation.
- Never criticize the self or allow negative thoughts to linger. Negativity produces a separation from the self, a split state of mind that prevents unity of purpose.
- When the mind wanders, return to focus on slow breathing.
- Stay in moment to moment reality, integrating the removal of obstacles as they pop up.
- Create clear visualizations of your intention. Include details of actions.

**Examples**

The monologue changes according to the focus of intention. When an effective pattern is found, continue to use key phrases and images that make it happen.

Lee Strasberg used inner-monologue training at Actor's Studio. This was back in the '60s and '70s in NYC. Enabling moment to moment performance, inner-monologue and relaxation are central to Method acting. At the time I had no idea it was also central to meditation techniques and living in the moment. I began to get the picture with Gurdjieff's famous *remember yourself* exercise in Ouspensky's *In Search of the Miraculous*.

Gurdjieff asked his students to run a moment by moment inner-monologue during the walk to class every morning. The purpose was to remember yourself and observe the immediate environment simultaneously. The difficulty lies in having to direct attention both towards the self (inner focus) and toward the object (outer focus) simultaneously.

The exercise required basic action in the following manner: *I step left, I right step, my arms swinging, I see this, I see that etc.* No one completed the exercise because there were endless distractions along the way. They would forget the objective and become involved in day dreams or street-side entertainment. Gurdjieff's students were top of the line mystics and yet they had major problems realizing the objective. Is it impossible to do? I don't think so and it sure is fun to practice an inner monologue on moment to moment realities. Include the observation of yourself doing whatever. Try to maintain the exercise from point a) to point b) and see what happens.

One morning, hiking in the forest I was meditating on just this problem in a slightly different context. It went like this – *how can I explain the technique of being totally relaxed and alert, almost vigilant, simultaneously?* I started practicing just in time to notice the very bushy tail of what quickly turned out to be a gorgeous coyote only a few feet from my little dogs. A coyote can snatch a small animal or lure one quickly into a trap in the flash of an eye. Their wily abilities are honored throughout the west. I quickly scooped up the pups and we moved on.

It's possible the appropriate inner monologue, quite by chance, saved the day. I was in a state of relaxed vigilance. Knowing my habit of monitoring the rough terrain under my feet – I could have missed the coyote a little above me, hidden in the scrub brush and trees. But the vigilance aspect of the monologue caused me to scan the environment.

There are more aspects of this exercise found in "Techniques of Consciousness Expansion."

*Don't allow the shadows*
*To put out the light;*
*Keep those campfires burning*
*Shining through the night.*

# Seeing Auras

The Aura is the glow of light emanating from the physical body and manifesting in a wide range of shapes and colors which indicate physical health and energy vibration. Illness produces an absence of light, causing a shadow around area under stress. Mystic Elizabeth Haich gives an excellent description of the absence of light in the illness she saw moving toward her sister's room in the memorable book *Initiation*.

"They were both full-size human forms, absolutely black like shadows........I did not really see these beings themselves but the hole they made in the rays of light where they were....They were shadows because of the complete absence of light."

A visible light radiates from all living creatures. Kirlian electro photography reveals basic light patterns of a subject. This technique of photography originated in Russia and was banned from the USA until the mid '70s. It was first presented (in America) at the Academy of Science in NYC and I was there. Hundreds of photo-slides were projected revealing electron/ion emissions from human subjects, trees, plants and animals under a myriad of conditions.

An interesting series of photos showed light-emissions of human subjects undergoing various forms of drug therapy. The bottom line was dramatic. Light patterns emanating from fingertips filled into a normal signature when the subject had appropriate drug for manifesting illness. Healthy subjects, given aspirin or psychotropic drugs, lost large sections of their light pattern. It looked like a short circuit occurred.

Another series of Kirlian photos showed a fountain of light shooting up from a tree at the moment of decapitation. I can still see it in my mind's eye. I wish someone would take Kirlian photos of folks using 4G phones and wireless devices. There would be stunning results.

Although the Kirlian evidence presented at the conference was totally convincing there is still enormous controversy regarding the actual process which is: a high-frequency charge is sent through a metal plate on a Polaroid film camera base. Fingertips or whatever are placed on the film, inside a black bag and the electric exposure is made.

Auras are influenced by philosophy of life and daily input, including nutrition, environment and mental focus. What goes in comes out at every level of expression. Sometimes what goes in doesn't get out. It's captured, so to speak, in the brain folds or the gut folds. In which case stagnation ensues and shadows begin to develop.

I recall the first time I saw a distinct shadow across a portion of someone's chest. There it was and I really didn't know what to think or say. Finally I asked if they had a history of heart disease and they said yes. I went on to learn it was a family disease – all family members had died from heart issues.

Shadows exist when energy is no longer circulating properly to an area; there is less light. This absence of light is the opposite of a glowing aura emitted by a healthy entity. Feelings of unconditional love can chase shadows away and stimulate a glow. The radiating light meditation found in the "Charisma" chapter is helpful.

My NYU students had great success with the radiating light practice in terms of seeing energy in classmates. And the observations confirmed the experiences of most participants. They could see *energy-suckers* as dark shadows with energy being drawn into the body and quickly dissipating while others were light radiators, almost glowing in the dark. The *radiating light* meditation created extreme wide-focus viewing which allowed for expanded perception.

Do you see *auras*? All living things radiate energy in the form of light patterns. *Seeing* is encouraged by relaxed, wide-focus viewing. The wide-focus switches attention away from *form* detection and toward *energy* detection. Empty the mind into no-thought and gaze at the person without expecting any results. Expect nothing. Result orientation pushes *the shining* away.

Why is the ability to see auras helpful in life? When *seeing* is accurate it gives one a reliable indicator of intentionality in others – as related in the following personal experience.

*Don't let the dogs out until that car leaves* my inner monologue stated as I pulled into the parking area at the trail head. So I waited for a few minutes, grew impatient and let out my Chihuahua who took off running in the general direction of a woman emerging from the bathroom facility. She was at enough distance I couldn't see details of her face. She leaned down, petted Bobo and picked her up at which point I saw a streak of light leave the side of her head and shoot toward the car a little distance away. I knew she intended to leave with my dog so I jogged toward her as she screamed in a raucous voice: "This is my dog and I'm taking her with me." We both arrived by the car at the same time and I was able to retrieve my precious animal.

The ability to see shadows created by waning or obstructed energy in the body can be most helpful in maintaining health in family members including animals. Which reminds me of a time in Georgia when I observed my treasured jackass approximately 5 acres in the distance and knew he was very ill. Although he was a silver-white color he looked like a very dark donkey. He had pneumonia.

Another source of light explosions is from the 7 chakras which are synonymous with the major nerve plexes of western medicine.

| Chakras | Affinities | Nerve Plexus | |
| --- | --- | --- | --- |
| Sahasrara (Crown) | Thought/Space | Pineal gland | Violet |
| Ajña (Third Eye) | Light/Dark | Carotid | Indigo |
| Vishuddhi (Throat) | Ether/Sound | Pharyngeal | Blue |
| Anahata (Heart) | Air | Cardiac | Green |
| Manipura (Navel) | Fire | Solar/Celiac | Yellow |
| Svadhisthana (Sacral) | Water | Splenic | Orange |
| MuladHara (Root) | Earth | Coccygeal | Red |

Chakras date back to ancient Buddhist texts written in Sanskrit and beyond to Mount Meru in Africa. A simple comparison of Chakras with major nerve plexes of western medicine reveals identical placement in the body. Some might wonder how the ancients could *see* what was later discovered in 16th Century dissected cadavers. Meditation made them good at energy detection.

Emotions affect Chakra centers radically, causing a release of little bursts of light with passionate feelings. Health issues produce varying degrees of murkiness in the chakra/plexus associated with illness underway. You must look with wide-focus to see these changes. Murky is the beginning of shadows.

Chakras are also control centers for energy exchange with *The Field* (prana), regulating changes in frequency and enabling expanded levels of consciousness. A study of chakras is a vast subject with many impressive documents written on the subject. If interested, I suggest starting with Charles Leadbeater and Hiroshi Motoyama.

The following quote from *The Chakras* by Leadbeater speaks of energy movement in what sounds identical to descriptions of the Field. "Astral matter, though so far finer than physical, is yet denser than that of the mental plane; the great clouds of "emotion forms" which are generated in the astral world by strong feelings do not all fly to one world-centre, but they do coalesce with other forms of the same nature in their own neighborhood, so that enormous and very powerful blocks of feeling are floating about almost everywhere, and a man may readily come into contact with them and be influenced by them."

Throughout Leadbeater's book are references to radiating emotion attracting "clouds" of emotion of the identical nature.; the reader should see similarities between the above description and other manuscripts discussing *prana* (Sanskrit) and the Field described as the fluid of life running through all things.

Barbara Brennan has investigated Auras and chakras quite thoroughly in her book *Hands of Light*. She uses a pendulum to create chakra readings with extremely detailed energy diagnosis. She's a master of the pendulum and her book is a must for anyone interested in the healing arts. She worked as a research scientist at NASA's Goddard Research Center before becoming a healer. Her academic credentials should please most left-brain skeptics.

*Your body is a mirror*
*Reflecting all you are*
*Radiate your light*
*Be a shining star.*

# Body Language

Alexander Lowen wrote in *Depression and the Body* that people affect their environment in a manner congruent with their individual behavior, providing information to outside viewers as to intentions, wellness, skills and general personality.

The body reveals everything regarding health, confidence, experience, character, motive and emotional resonance (personal history). Every aspect of physical expression has meaning and can be read by observers. Our concern here is with body language that dramatically affects moment to moment reality.

Don't cover chakras (energy centers). Folding the arms over the chest covers the *solar plexus*, a major center for information exchange, and interferes with one's reading of outgoing and incoming frequencies. Crossing the legs and/or tightening the anus muscles cover the *muladHara chakra*, controls sexual energy and interferes with diaphragmatic breathing and relaxation. Covering the *heart chakra* with the arms or rounded shoulders reveals chronic fear of emotional expression. It interferes with intuition and allows muscles around the heart to become stiff, affecting the general health of the heart.

## Body Language

*Poor me* slumps into the lower-back with head tilted or protruded several inches in front of the body. Tilting the head is a behavior exhibited by some women when conversing with males. It shows deference to the male. Dropping the head or looking down while conversing is another way of showing deference. Both actions can produce feelings of subservience. Interestingly, animals also use the dropped head behavior to show subjugation to a dominant animal.

The *top-heavy pushover* – 'chest out, belly in' - *carries* body weight in the chest and shoulders. The lower body is usually stiff, particularly the legs. The pushover is prone to all types of accidents. Durckheim writes about the pushover in *Hara: The Vital Center of Man*. "Do you see that the Europeans standing here could be easily toppled over if one were suddenly to give them a little push from behind? But none of the Japanese would lose their balance even if they were given a much harder push." This is because the Japanese carry their center in the pelvic (Hara) region instead of the upper chest.

The *giggler* laughs before and/or after every verbal communication. It's a sign of insecurity and serves as a form of self-erasure. Gigglers are unaware of the habit and find it difficult to recognize even when pointed out. Oriental Medicine says regular giggling indicates heart strain and suggests a congenital problem.

The *figiter* expresses restlessness in constant movement by playing with objects, swinging a leg or drumming a foot while seated. The figiter experiences internal pressure from tension; movement postpones encountering the overwhelming feeling of exploding from within. Situations that prohibit emotional expression magnify behavior.

**Super-tight, sucked in lips** indicates a chronic breath holder. Usually these are tight-ass folks who maintain control over emotional expression. They are also frequently ill with flu and bacterial infections because they grab hold and don't release the disease.

Other relevant body language includes the many signs of contraction in the face, upper torso, leg and foot placement, balance and breath. All these qualities reveal long term tensions and/or short term discomfort.

Incessant talking is often a cover-up for insecurities and inabilities in professional settings. This was true in various situations where those who spoke the loudest, with criticisms of other musicians couldn't keep time for the length of a tune. Same was true in a multitude of settings auditioning actors, prospective students and prospective teachers.

Body language configures the body in ways that affect us totally. If you are folded in on yourself with slumped, rounded shoulders and arms obscuring the solar-plexus then you are creating the same dynamic internally.

### Exercises

- Tune into the body language of others; it will increase ability to recognize signature expressions in yourself.
- Practice keeping the body in a neutral state as defined in earlier chapters.

- Observe body language dynamics in various situations and recognize who and what cause one to cover the solar plexus with folded arms, thereby creating a wall of separation. Covering the solar plexus is a popular behavior as you will observe. Often this covering indicates mistrust of something in the environment be it a person or a situation. It can become a habit hard to break.
- The ultimate experience of body language is experienced in a well known process known as *mirroring* in which one becomes the mirror image of the person one is in interaction with. It sounds as though the other would know they are being imitated –but not so. It has been found to make for more effective communication and greater rapport.

One experiences similar emotions as the one who is mirrored; to the point of seeing what the mirrored other is seeing. Keep in mind mirror dynamics: if the other picks up a cup with the left hand then pick your cup up with the right hand. When they lean to the left – you lean to the right and so on. Strangely enough, no one ever catches on to what is happening and it seems to put folks at ease and provide insight as to mood and intentionality.

*Santa Clause is just as real*
*As the CIA*
*If that's what you believe.*

# Visualize Paradise

Biofeedback studies reveal the power of the visual cortex to effect brain-wave frequencies and heart rate. Mental images impact every cell in the body and change the structure of the brain. We experience all visual events as though we lived through them.

We can learn to control brain-wave patterns, blood pressure and heart-beat with pleasurable visual input. Even lab rats can change heart rate to avoid administered shocks. Whatever we envision is what we create: Our images are self-fulfilling prophecies as life-experiences design mental and physical health.

**The placebo effect has proven belief over-powers biology**; the body can't distinguish between the mental and the physical because they are the same. One out of three patients taking a placebo improved; the person's belief changed the symptoms.

Negative states, particularly anger and depression are known to influence the development of illness whereas positive thinking heals disease and influences the outcome of everything one does. The evidence is overwhelming: positive thinking offers a longer, healthier, happier life.

Nobel Prize winning physicist Eugene Wiger states in *Space, Time and Medicine* by Larry Dossey MD: "If mind could not affect the physical world but was only affected by it, this would be the only known example in modern physics of such a one-way interaction. For in modern physics, one-way interactions are not known to occur."

What is negativity? Should we follow advice of chronic well wishers – *if you haven't something positive to say, say nothing at all.* If all negativity ceased it would be a quieter world: churches, news media and the arts would fall strangely silent along with power brokers at all levels of society.

Intention determines the dynamic of a negative attitude. If one's purpose is to encourage change for the betterment of a situation it will have a radically different impact than gossip, ill intentions and criticism of people, places and situations. When statements come from dedicated whistle blowers or support belief in action that creates hope for the future, they should not be considered negative.

Personal negativity, as expressed in gloomy inner-monologues, is damaging because darkness attracts darkness and so on. The *birds of a feather* are at it again. We attract and communicate with energies on our frequency band. Therefore it's good to run a positive inner-monologue whether we feel it or not. The inner monologue serves to instruct the mind/body to make corrections toward a more positive state of being.

Most negativity reflects a lack of self control, expressed through loose lips in a manner warned against in the numerous texts presented in "Listening." Idle chatter is a difficult habit to control; egos are soothed and pumped-up by the sound of one's voice.

Masaru Emoto's water books offer undeniable evidence of the incredible power of words on the structure of water. Since we are 90% water it behooves us to communicate *love and gratitude* particularly when the whistle-blower effect is under way.

You are probably familiar with the *laws of attraction* as presented in the popular film and book, *The Secret*, released in 2006. People tried to jump start their careers and finances by making posters representing objects of desire and placing them within sight. In order for this strategy to work, one's thoughts would need to support the premise of one's desires. My response to *The Secret* enthusiasts is usually "How is it working for you?" Because if it works by creating more joy and love – that is all that matters.

**Exercises**
- Should you catch yourself being verbally judgmental, critical, and pessimistic, stop and say aloud: *Please excuse me for this outburst of negativity. It's a state of being I'm working to remove from my expression. Let's find something positive and inspiring to discuss.*
- Instead of counting sheep, methodically recall the day's experiences in terms of positive expression. If you recall sleeping through outbursts of negativity then pursue the goal with greater objectivity. For example, make little one word notes or riddles and post them wherever you express yourself verbally. I started out with large posters and expanded into a painting illustrating the World War 2 admonition: "Loose lips sink ships."
- In extremely painful grief, the brain has the habit of running the experience non-stop. To master the obsessed mind is a primary objective of all self-healing and moves consciousness light-years closer to the truth.

- Visualize what you want. Stay in touch with your dreams by running positive images and positive dialogue in your inner monologue.
- Visualize a job interview with the bottom line: a job offer. Speak silently to interviewer as follows. *I am just the person you are looking for. I will expand sales and contribute to the creative impulse of Daisy Inc.* Turn on the *radiating light* as you walk through the door.
- Whenever negative tape-loops are running, visualize the positive outcome desired. Observe the effect positive visualization has on all circumstances.
- Don't communicate fear and criticism to children. Give them images of love, success, good health and hope for the future.
- Avoid media violence and negativity for a week. Do you feel better in general? Are you less fearful?
- Balance emotional pain with positive experiences. Often it's necessary to force oneself to have a good time. Watch a funny movie during period of grief or depression.
- Practice positive actions. It doesn't matter how you feel. Pretense transforms into reality. Act to move one small step closer to achieving an important goal. Acting on positive thoughts enriches personal freedom.
- Make it a game to abstain from unproductive communication. When close friends and relatives habitually express negativity, involve them in your process.
- Avoid sado-masochistic relationships. When someone repeatedly makes you unhappy, it's time to drop the relationship. The first time a mate strikes you, move on immediately. There is never an excuse for hurting a loved one and the abuse will reoccur. It's guaranteed.
- Keep a record of the evolution and outcome of positive-thinking that move you to undreamed of opportunity.

It's easy to lose contact with yourself and wakeup years later wondering where you've been. Quality solitude allows one to review activities, make plans, and redirect negativity into a glorious paradise.

The bottom line is, we are what we believe. If you believe in prayer it will work for you. If you believe in science the same holds true. Whatever you wish to accomplish, focus on it and push the button for the desired frequency to enable arrival. Visualize paradise.

# Part Two

# Expanding Consciousness

*Why use one
When you have two?
The right is for dreaming
The left is for scheming.*

# Bimodal Consciousness

The ongoing dialectic between the two brain hemispheres can be a source of stress and confusion when the two hemispheres are at odds with each other. During periods of critical decision making, one hemisphere is urging the opposite of what the other hemisphere wants. Sound familiar? The argument is intensified when habitual response favors one brain over the other, without awareness of the moment's demands.

This is particularly true for psychic awareness which is seated in the right brain (RB). Left brain (LB) dominants such as economists, mathematicians and computer geeks tend to suppress RB capabilities which encompass techniques and inclinations that take one beyond ordinary reality. **It's impossible to explore the unknown when focused on rules and regulations.**

Most LB science doesn't recognize the more esoteric approach to healing such as acupuncture, shiatsu, radionics, yoga, meditation and preventive medicine and RB artistic types are often judged as strange, living on the fringe of society and out of touch with the so-called real world.

The following dichotomies are used to describe two separate modes of consciousness, one associated with each hemisphere of the brain. Maintaining a balance between the two brains affects all aspects of physical and mental expression. The terms listed below describe focus, process and method of each hemisphere.

| Right Brain (RB) | Left Brain (LB) |
|---|---|
| Sub-conscious | Conscious |
| Eastern thought | Western thought |
| Expansion | Contraction |
| Yin | Yang |
| Left side of body | Right side |
| Emotional | Rational |
| Spatial, visual | Verbal |
| Sensuous, intuitive | Intellectual |
| Representational | Abstract |

| | |
|---|---|
| Essence | Origin |
| Inner directed (alpha) | Outer Directed (Beta) |
| Space | Time |
| Inductive (whole to part) | Deductive (part to whole) |
| Paradox | Logic |
| Reactive (receptive) | Manipulative |
| Physical | Mental |
| Nouns, adjectives | Verbs, predicates |
| Diffuse, divergent | Focused, discrete |
| Sign (motive) | Symbol |
| Magnetic | Electric |
| Introvert | Extrovert |
| Wide-focus | Narrow-focus |
| India | America |
| Feminine | Masculine |
| Artistic | Scientific |
| Earth | Air |
| Roots | Branches |
| Unconventional | Cautious |
| Impulse | Discipline |
| Bright colors | Gray, black, white |
| Submissive | Dominant |
| Dark | Light |
| Cold | Hot |
| Magnesium | Calcium |
| Yielding | Resistance |
| Melody | Rhythmic articulation |

Bimodal consciousness refers to brain hemispheres working together in harmony. Harmony means both hemispheres receive input without conflict and use the method appropriate for the situation. Piaget outlines a bimodal dialectic as the creative process; his four stages of development reveal a productive harmony between the two hemispheres.

- Preparation: techniques, education, training, research, practice (LB)
- Incubation: Turning things over to the subconscious mind (RB)
- Illumination: The Eureka moment when left-brain material is given form by the right brain or vice-versa. (Bimodal)
- Verification: does it work? (Bimodal)

The bimodal process involves the coming together of opposites. Right-brained skills such as imagination, emotion and visual processing are shaped by left-brain focus, detail, research and organization. The two modes working together produce insight, content, meaning and direction.

Illumination occurs as one is able to experience, to invent, to develop imaginative dichotomies. The dichotomies should be one from each brain. For example, refined technique and extreme passion, or performing a high-tension task in a relaxed, slow beta frequency.

Mindfulness, remembering-yourself, yin/yang and other techniques designed to expand consciousness involve the synthesis of opposites. These techniques demand right-brain dominance with oversight of the left-hemisphere. This is an approach rarely considered in formal education where left-brain dominance agitates against RB processing. Even to the extreme of removing the arts from school curriculums.

When choosing a school for one's children, remember the importance of the arts. It is about more than learning how to paint, dance, play an instrument or write creatively. It is about a mode of consciousness that enriches every aspect of life. It is about the essence of how one sees the world.

In general, the LB represses the irrational and guards against the intrusion of alien feelings, as illustrated in the following chapter. Or the RB does not wish to be bothered by annoying details or pedestrian analysis. Listen closely and you can hear the two brains in discussion inside your head, in politics, in personal relationships and throughout society. Democrat and Republican dialectics personify the process as witnessed in the debt-ceiling debate. Our political parties represent the extremes of LB/RB processing.

A comparison of India and America gives an excellent visualization of the dichotomy between the two modes of consciousness. Memories of India go back to the '80s when I made a solo, 3 month visit to the land of many wonders. Upon arrival, my first destination was the bank, to get some rupees. It was a mind blower; there was no filing system or apparent organization what-so-ever. At the largest bank in Delhi files were stacked up against the wall, towering close to the ceiling in great disarray. Not too much different from the luggage pick-up area at the airport. My red backpack was at the top of an enormous, 16' pile of luggage thrown in the corner: I had to climb to the top to retrieve it.

Yet in the smallest towns, shabby looking book stores held great treasures on shelves stacked with metaphysical books from most cultures, particularly in the area of philosophy and the healing arts. Ragged urchin types could be seen hunkered down reading serious looking volumes as they awaited patrons to their sidewalk business. The country that brought us the Buddha, meditation and yoga is an example of RB dominant, bimodal consciousness. Basically they handle the material world in a RB mode, while their metaphysical preoccupations demonstrate much discipline for LB word processing and focus.

Intuition is a RB dominant expression which can show signs of paranoia when unaccompanied by LB rationality, questioning input with "Where do you think this impulse is coming from? Is it an initiator or a reaction?" You will be surprised by the answers that return from the inquiry.

Writing in *Future Memory*, P.M.H. Atwater mentions a third category of brain processing, the Limbic System, which she says is "the gateway and guide to superconscious, synergistic aspects of awareness." This path to super consciousness is approached through the RB, making RB dominance primary to expanding awareness beyond our limited perceptions.

The Limbic System (LS) is called the center of feelings and is considered the main provider of motivational context, attention control and memory management. Why would this be of interest to our inner-journey? Emotions are linked to the RB, and the LS is the seat of emotions – making the RB connection with the LS stronger than the LB connection. The LS is where pre-conscious awareness is initiated and that is our destination, making RB dominance essential to our journey. If you are LB dominant, change is called for to live a more creative, inspired life full of meaning, passion and insight.

Knowing one's dominant hemisphere will avoid fighting natural inclination in terms of training and job preference. A RB consciousness will rarely flourish in an office environment full of rules & regulations and sequential processing. Whereas, LB folks feel ill at ease in unstructured environments. Bimodal embraces the best of both worlds.

*Where are we going?*
*What will we find?*
*Live in the moment,*
*Forget about time.*

# A Cautionary Tale

In the summer of 2001 a very dear friend and business associate came to NM to visit; I hadn't seen him for 19 years. The man I had known was highly creative, receptive with incredible imagination and a delightful sense of humor, far from the uptight, rigid man who appeared at my door.

I recognized something radical had changed in his personality as we began planning a trip to Chaco Canyon the morning after his arrival. He wanted to look at maps and plan the trip; I told him I had been there 3 times and could almost make the trip with eyes closed, but he insisted on plotting every turn (**LB**). In fact he became upset when I suggested we just take it as it came along (**RB**).

We had a half tank of gas as we reached Angel Fire, a small mountain town with a gas station. I suggested filling up, explaining we may not have the opportunity further west. He was driving and insisted we had sufficient gas for the moment and could get some later. I have yet to understand why he was so dogmatically insistent, but he came to regret it as the 2nd half of the trip became a frantic search for gas with the meter on empty.

Finally we arrived at Chaco around 5pm and he drove directly to the bulletin board to see the rules and regulations (**LB**). I suggested that first we needed to check out the few remaining camp sites available but no, off he went to learn what we could and could not do. He came back to the car and said my little dogs would have to be on leases at all times (**LB**). I said no, we would go moment to moment and if the need arose I would act accordingly (**RB**).

We found a site where he could set up his tent; I would be sleeping in the car and remained there taking photos until shortly after sunset when the heavy bug population retired for the evening (**RB**). He stayed very busy with this and that – arranging things in particular orders, seemingly oblivious to hundreds of stingers all around him (**LB**).

Moments before sunset we were having a cup of tea in the crowded camping arena when I looked up at the sky directly above to see one of the most memorable sights of a life time. The entire sky was filled with a slow moving vortex of identically shaped clouds, flat on the bottom with 3 large scallops on the top, moving clockwise into the vortex, with the largest clouds on the outside. The clouds became smaller and smaller as they drew nearer the center. It was so uniform that it looked computer generated.

I looked around to see if the other campers were watching and saw everybody was busy cooking and eating and nobody was looking up (**RB**). I looked at my companion and he was oblivious like everyone else – so I tapped him on the shoulder and pointed up. His mouth fell open in amazement.

At the time I reasoned that if energy vortexes of this nature occurred with frequency at Chaco, it made sense why the Anasazi Indians chose this remote, brutally hot and cold desert location to build a spiritual center for all tribes. Later as I learned more about HAARP I figured they must have been conducting sky-maneuvers in the NM deserts once again. Whatever the case, it was truly awesome.

When we arrived back in Taos a friend was at the house; the three of us had tea as I told her about the event. My Chaco companion chimed in saying "consider the source" (**LB**). At which point I stopped the story, saying I'd tell her later.

At dinner I asked if he had seen the vortex over our heads. He replied that he had seen it. Then I asked why he had made the statement "consider the source." And he replied: "Because it was so way out, I had no place to put it" (**LB**). I responded: "Why do you have to put it anywhere" (**RB**)?

In the course of 19 years he had moved from a highly creative life (**RB**) to one as an administrative director (**LB**). I guess for some it would be considered a more prestigious professional position and to be sure the pay was much better but he had lost contact with his excellent awareness, creative consciousness and zany personality.

A lack of Bimodal consciousness supports a one track mind which can be caught by surprise around every corner. Or perhaps one is oblivious of what is happening in the immediate environment. Folks who cannot see an amazing vortex filling the sky above them might also be unaware of everything else going on around them. And if they did notice something, would they pretend to have seen nothing (**LB**)?

When one is tuned into an objective universal consciousness it offers guidance of a balanced and productive nature. The inner voice might whisper, *you are missing something* or *extremism is blocking your view*. Over time one develops sensitivity to balance and truth that will insist on expression as consciousness.

The repeating loop of daily routine may exclude awareness of realities underway such as preparations for control of the masses by use of microwave grids throughout the country, resigning of the Patriot Act by a president who promised change, representatives that seem to have forgotten separation of church and state and anti-Robin Hood enrichment of the very source of the world-wide economic crisis. Without awareness we cannot create the change so desperately needed to manifest peace in the world. It's important to know what is going on in one's community, which is usually a mirror of the national zeitgeist.

Be sure to read "Zapping the Masses" in the Appendix.

*Lead the way; Save the day*
*From rules and regulations.*
*They stultify & nullify*
*Our lives and inspirations.*

# Increasing Right Brain Dominance

The objective of this book is to increase awareness, expand consciousness and become proficient at extra-sensory perception and creative processing. Therefore most of the practices are of a RB nature and increase the function of that mode of consciousness.

In today's world, particularly since the 9/11 event and the wireless revolution, we are inundated with LB strategies, techniques and mode of consciousness. Western education has always focused on training the LB and basically ignoring the RB but now we have further excluded the RB by cutting music, art, physical education, art history and drama from the classroom while increasing hours staring at computer and TV screens in the home environment.

Basically we spend a lot of time sitting on our duffs living our lives through the TV. Consider removing it to an inaccessible room and engaging in activities that do not involve electrical devices. Bet that's a scary thought! But one doesn't want the home to be an extension of the LB work and school environment. Make your home a RB haven.

Teaching for 7 years in alphabet city on the lower east side of NYC was a challenge. The children came from unusual home situations and had to move past drug dealers and burned out structures every morning. We made their life experience a part of our classroom process. An example of a standing assignment was to write about what they saw on the way to school every morning. We also made maps of the neighborhood and conducted door to door surveys regarding on-going events and on and on. Every child had a camera donated by Kodak and we put them to great use. There was never a lack of opportunity to encourage RB expression.

The proof of success was their enthusiasm. They were waiting for my arrival in the morning, screaming Odin, Odin as I rode up on my bicycle. They returned early after lunch and consistently turned in homework. We were never consumed with rules and regulations; in fact there was only one rule: Do not hurt another child mentally or physically. We passed all the State quiz's while maintaining a RB classroom environment.

Some educators fail to encourage Bimodal consciousness or make the student central to the learning process by focusing skills toward subjects of interest. The Rudolph Steiner Waldorf Schools allow the child's imagination to be the guide and encourage RB development and expression to the fullest. It is the best possible education a child can experience. Steiner was an outstanding humanitarian, mystic and recognized enemy by Adolph Hitler.

The first grade can be difficult for boys because LB skills develop later than girls, making the 3 Rs difficult to comprehend unless taught in a RB manner. Schools are often too ready to label a child with a learning disability – instead of creating a learning experience with personal images and less abstraction.

Kindergarten and Elementary School classrooms are filled with children hunting and pecking wireless, 4G MW antenna devices toward intellectual inferiority. 4G devices were recently introduced as tools of education in kindergarten. How can anything be more LB dominant, not to mention the effect of MW frequency on concentration and the immune system.

In *Public Health SOS; The Shadow Side of the Wireless Revolution* Magda Havas and Camilla Rees have written about the extreme effect wireless has on very young children which includes the high level of radiation penetrating their softer skulls and numerous health effects.

Parents concerned with possibilities inherent to LB dominant education might want to try some of the following strategies to increase RB dominance.

## Techniques

- Reduce use of wireless in the home such as play stations and other wireless devices.
- Use computers for research and composition instead of playtime.
- Focus on physical activities after school such as sports, gym, martial arts and dance.
- Reduce TV viewing; short segments of content between ads make it a LB tool.
- Encourage family to draw. Use *Drawing on the Right Side of the Brain* by Betty Edwards to develop skills. Throughout the book she relates to everything in terms of LB/RB. For the most part she encourages turning the LB off.
- Improve pattern recognition with books like *Yoga for the Brain* by Sandy Steen Bartholomew. It's a project for all ages.
- Keep a journal about emotional feelings – no facts – just feelings.
- Join a theatre group. Drama is very RB.

- Seek out and be receptive to unfamiliar information.
- When conversing listen for RB clues such as inflection, tone of voice, facial expression and body language. The LB is only concerned with the literal meaning of words.
- Create physical exercises using the left side of the body only. Jump on the left leg while moving the left hand and arm. This immediately moves one into the RB; this is due to contralateral processing.
- Dreams are the RB pathway to the subconscious. (Electrical stimulation of the RB creates a dreamlike state full of emotional, non-verbal images.) As you drift off to sleep focus on where you wish to go in your dreams and what you would like to learn. Keep a pad and pencil nearby to write down what dreams may come before they escape.
- Sit in the morning before beginning your day and hum a favorite melody very slowly, holding each note at least 3 beats and breathing diaphragmatically, to be followed by a few seconds of either false or real laughter. It will work wonders.
- Drinking dulls the RB more than the LB whereas marijuana does the opposite.
- Rap and Heavy Metal are LB; they focus on rhythm and are often devoid of melody whereas melodic music is highly RB. Singing, chanting and humming moves one into the RB. Chanting has been used to upgrade consciousness since before the PHaraohs ruled.
- As mentioned earlier, color is associated with the RB. If you are extremely LB force yourself to wear color and unusual styles. Aversion to wearing bright colors is a testament to your hemisphere preference.
- Involve children in projects to assist the poor and under-privileged, particularly during holiday seasons. Compassion and empathy are to be encouraged as RB qualities needed in the world today as never before.
- Encouraging intuition and other paranormal abilities calls for quieting the ongoing instruction/criticism from the verbal LB. The easiest way to quiet verbal consciousness is to focus on counted breathing and /or singing a song. You will find it impossible to maintain an inner dialogue and focus on these activities simultaneously.

- Don't take young boys hunting. Children, particularly under thirteen years, have a strong affinity with animals. It breaks their hearts to kill creatures they love and deeply identify with. It will cause them to avoid RB emotions in order to handle their heartbreak.
- Encourage children to express emotions.

*Where is your balance?*
*You're not in bed.*
*Walk on your feet*
*Not on your head.*

# Balancing Act

Zen philosophy advocates moderation or the *middle-way* as the path of action. Throughout the *Tao Teh King,* Lao Tzu consuls: "avoid extremes, shunning excess in one way as well as in the other.....one who acts naturally avoids extremes." This is true for body, mind and soul; severe imbalance reflects across the entire spectrum of well being. All input affects output particularly in the areas of nutrition, exercise, sensory stimulation and frequency exchange.

Most readers have heard of homeostasis which is the ability of an organism or cell to maintain internal balance by adjusting physiological processes. Homeostasis is dedicated to maintaining body temperature, pH balance and blood glucose levels. Poor nutrition radically impacts homeostasis, creating some of the most dreaded diseases.

**Nutrition**

Nutrition, a vast and complicated subject, isn't given a required course of study in medical school. According to several friends who attended Emory University back in the '80s, not one word was mentioned about nutrition. Now they are psychiatrics dispensing anti-depressants and other meds as cure alls. The same holds true for veterinarians – known to recommend poisonous diets and often paid to promote the poorest food brands. Rarely does either group makes recommendations regarding nutrition as a preventive measure or as a possible solution.

Meanwhile, the chemistry of the body is greatly affected by the amount of sugar, carbs and saturated fat eaten. According to Nora Gedgaudas (certified nutritional therapist and neurofeedback specialist and author of *Primal Body, Primal Mind*) sugar and carbs are the primary causes of mental and physical disease and should be avoided. Whereas saturated fat and cholesterol, when consumed in the absence of sugar and carbs, are necessary for optimal mental health.

Gedgaudas suffered from depression for 35 years before diet and neurofeedback gave back her life for the past 15 years. A healthy biochemistry = healthier emotions; she will make you want to be a fat burner instead of a sugar burner, using a system not unlike the Atkin's diet and Suzanne Somers' system.

*"Mental Illness Surveillance Among Adults in the US"*, a 9/11 report from the Center for Disease Control says at minimum – ¼ of the population suffers from mental illness. They go on to say there is more mental illness in developing countries than any illness including heart disease and cancer.

Gedgaudas points out the USDA estimates the average person consumes 12 teaspoons of sugar daily. Did you know Alzheimer's disease often comes to those with an extreme sweet tooth? Not good! She also reiterates a well known admonition: *eat less; calorie restriction will greatly lengthen your life.* This information is confirmed by many sources and should be welcome in our current economy. Read her important book *Primal Body, Primal Mind: Beyond the Paleo Diet for Total Health and Longer Life* for stunning details.

Many years ago I wrote on the blackboard in my 4th grade classroom "You are what you eat!" When we returned to the room after lunch some enterprising student had written under the quote "Eat the teacher." Fairly humorous reply with no ill will intended – but did they get the message? It's a message requiring research, constant modification and an iron will.

## Physical Balance

Physical balance is necessary to avoid all manner of injury, particularly relevant for the athlete and the elderly. It is rooted in the Hara with the bulls-eye two inches below the navel. Martial arts exercises are designed to pull the *chi* energy into the Hara and establish this abdominal area as the center of all movement. The Tanden (bulls eye) is the seat of that power known as *one point*; when one stands with bent knees and breaths into the Tanden one feels balanced and powerful. The purpose of the Wing Chun exercise mentioned earlier is to establish contact with this powerhouse.

Balance removes the inclination to contract which pulls one out of the Hara and away from the feet – the two platforms of balance. It's much harder to fall into holes, slip from ladders, stumble over obstructions or slip in the tub when balanced, making it an important objective for the accident prone.

When executing Wing Chun stance with knees touching, one feels incredible power as the feet spread out against the floor like pancakes and the chi drops into the Hara. When one allow the muscles to push upward the entire body trembles like a leaf in a storm and balance is gone.

The *I Ching* or *Book of Changes* is a great source for considering the metaphysical aspects of balance. It is a source of prophesy with the emphasis on change and balance and contains much wisdom regarding dynamic equilibrium of opposites as aspects of the whole, as in two sides of the mountain, both sides of the coin, good/bad, in/out – one could not exist without the other. Or as Helmet Wilhelm writes in *Eight Lectures on the I Ching* "….everything absolute and unconditional already implies its own death." Meaning: avoid extremes.

"All work and no play make Jack a dull boy." And the reverse is equally true. It's important to maintain an apparent balance in activity, behavior and focus. Extremes are to be avoided which usually means working to overcome natural inclinations. This pursuit is aided by the *remember yourself* and *moment to moment* practices.

Hopefully personal balance will eventually encourage fairness in government, where manipulated chaos and obvious extremes are rampant. As Talbot Mundy writes in *Om, the Secret of Arbor Valley*, we have the government we deserve. That is certainly an indictment of our age where government bestows great riches on the wealthiest while depriving the middle class, poor and elderly. When will we see through elegant, self-serving words and elect representatives that desire balanced realities for the majority?

**Exercises for Physical Balance**
- Meditate on the *Hara*, breathing slowly into the area and imagine it expanding until the entire body is radiating light.
- Plant feet firmly on the ground, shoulder width apart with the knees bent. With focus on *Tanden*, repeat ten to 20 times: *one point* while tapping at the *Tanden* level with fingers gathered together into a point.
- Release the weight in the upper body onto to the feet. Feel the feet expand as they receive the body weight. There should be equal weight on both feet. Maintain a straight spine from the head to the tail-bone.
- When energy jumps into the upper body, grip the floor with the toes. Repeat the phrase **one point.** Let go of the muscles at the pelvic floor while keeping the lumbar section of the back tucked under. The feet are expanded noticeably against the floor. Breathe diaphragmatically.

Before doing this exercise have a partner, standing in front of you, gently push on your shoulders and chest in attempt to knock you off balance. After doing the *one point* exercise, try the pushing by a partner again and note the improvement. In time you should be able to hold your position easily.

- Shake and stretch your legs until they feel loose. Stand with knees bent a little and determine if both legs feel the same in terms of weight, internal consistency, tightness and looseness. Massage the problem leg and use acupressure on tight muscles until both legs feel the same.
- Never stand, walk or jump with straight knees. Tuck the rear under slightly and move from the pelvis. Don't stand on one leg or shift back and forth between the legs. Standing on one leg indicates a weakness on the opposite side of the body.
- Walk, stand, sit and perform movements in front of a mirror and observe symmetry. Make the two sides mirror images of each other.
- Shiatsu, Tai Chi, Yoga, Alexander-techniques focus on balance and centering energy. Classes of this nature produce results for readers who can't discipline themselves to work alone.
- Refer to Alan North's *The Urban Adventure Handbook* for advanced balancing techniques used in loose-chain-walking and rock/wall climbing.
- Stand on one leg, lift the other leg with the knee raised waist high. Maintain the position without wobbling. Sink body weight into the standing foot. Sometimes one leg maintains better balance than the other, indicating imbalance on that side.
- To test balance, jump high into the air and land on one leg with the raised knee waist high. Hold the position for a few seconds before jumping to the other leg. Sing or make sound with a strong voice while jumping from leg to leg. Practice until it becomes easy. Go easy with all exercise to the degree of proficiency in order to avoid injury of some sort.
- Physical balance reveals a lot about internal well-being. Imbalance suggests one side of the body is experiencing itself as denser, heavier, stiffer, softer or tighter. Remember we subconsciously withdraw energy (electrical current) from an area that is chronically ill, painful or coming down with a problem.

*Balance extremes and*
*Live out your dreams*
*Nothing can stop you.*

# According to Yin and Yang

The concept of Yin and Yang is concerned with the movement of energy between two extremes. Ideas surrounding this concept developed from observation and discovering pairs of mutually independent opposites that give meaning to each other. For example, *up* has little meaning without *down*.

Yin is the tendency toward expansion and Yang, the tendency toward contraction. There is constant movement between these extremes. The Chinese experience this exchange as central to Chinese Medicine and martial arts.

Opposites are eternally evolving and recycling through transformations, balance, interaction and dependant opposition. All phenomena turn into their opposite in the yin-yang philosophy of balance and continual change. Western philosophy has a strong tendency to experience a more static either-or nature such as right-wrong, black-white and in-out.

The philosophy of Yin and Yang is a mysterious and often misunderstood subject with major ramifications in daily life. The understanding here is focused on the quality and quantity of energy available and the maintenance of acid (-) and alkaline (+) balance essential for good health.

Extreme Yang indicates too much energy and extreme Yin, too little energy. Extreme yang type people are thin with tight, hard muscles, aggressive, angular and stiff movements with frequent insomnia and chronic digestive problems. The extreme yin type is unmotivated, withdrawn and overweight with soft, flaccid muscle tone. They may live in a fantasy world or experience chronic depression.

An extreme yin condition (kyo) feels soft to the fingers. The fingers sink into the area a little too far. Jitsu is an extreme yang condition of too much energy and feels hard and pushing back to the fingers. A jitsu area is easier to treat with shiatsu, massage and finger stimulation whereas kyo requires continual modification to return the energy to the area of concern. Kyo indicates a more serious condition.

How does one know their condition? Some indications of Yin imbalance are a tendency to feel cold, depression, abdominal bloating, retention of fluids, feeling of heaviness and puffy eyes and face. Asparagus, kale, fish, green tea, turnips and basmati rice are considered helpful in returning to greater balance.

Yang imbalance expresses as restless sleep, easily stressed/irritated, constipation, dry skin, feeling too warm in hot weather, very talkative, headaches, fever blisters and canker sores. The yang person needs cooling foods such as salads, spinach, melons, sushi and non-spicy dishes.

A reoccurring theme at the Cancer Dialogue in NYC was the acid/alkaline balance of the body. Cancer experts from all over the world discussed chronic extreme acidity as the proven precancerous environment. Bottom line: cancer has a hard time developing in a highly alkaline environment.

Cancer is not the only energy that thrives in an acid environment. Medical statistics claim most people over the age of 55 have digestive problems. Irritable bowel syndrome is a major, chronic, and difficult to cure condition that should be approached more from the perspective of balancing the potential hydrogen (pH) in the body. The pH measures the number of (-) hydroxyl ions which are alkaline forming as opposed to the amount of hydrogen (H+) ions that are acid forming. An easy way to get an indication of your internal balance is with diagnostic pH test strips. The *"pH ion Balance"* strips are considered one of the best for measuring acid/alkaline in the urine and saliva with a 6.4 pH considered the best reading.

Dr. Baroody writes in *Alkalize or Die*,"....pH is the measurement of electrical resistance between negative and positive ions in the body." The action between the two creates one's electro-chemical signature. Alkaline forming minerals are: Magnesium, Potassium, Iron, and Manganese.

When living on a ranch I monitored the bowel movements of my animals closely – with the exception of the cattle, in which case it's hard to modify their grass diet in the case of diarrhea. The grains and grasses eaten by cattle are acidic; their poop is extremely loose indicating an acidic condition. Is it any wonder meat is acidic?

Bowel movements of my donkeys, mules, dogs and cats always indicated the condition of their health. An example is my elderly jackass who had extremely small, dry, ball shaped stool. I hand fed him a more alkaline mush and the condition improved.

### Application and Exercise

Meditate on the following categories and determine if you have balanced yin and yang. The lists are used for identification and guidance in creating ongoing harmonic exchange. Experiment with diet and exercise to moderate imbalance. Baroody's book contains an extensive list of foods, minerals and supplements with their acid/alkaline values.

| YIN | YANG |
|---|---|
| Matter | Energy |
| Darkness | Light |
| Female | Male |
| Expansion | Contraction |
| Alkaline | Acidic |
| Inhalation | Exhalation |
| Cold | Hot |
| Right-brain | Left-brain |
| Sleep | Alertness |
| Stillness | Movement |
| Face: oblong, triangular, pale | Red, round or square |

| Alkaline Producing Foods | Acid Producing Foods |
|---|---|
| Cantaloupe | Blueberries |
| Dates | Cranberries |
| Figs | Prunes |
| Asparagus | All rice, oats, wheat |
| Bee pollen | Most nuts |
| Lemons & grapefruit | Meat |

*Remember Jack and Jill*
*Humpty Dumpty too*
*Forget to bend your knees*
*The same will come to you*

# Avoiding Falls

Balance is achieved through body alignment, a low center of gravity, diaphragmatic breathing and bending knees. With these techniques in place one can encounter all manner of surprise experiences and arrive unbroken.

Balance needs to be second nature before reaching elderly years when life-threatening falls are known to increase. A survey conducted by orthopedic surgeons found over 150,000 falls recorded in the United States every year. 20,000 are serious and require surgery and long term treatment. This doesn't include sports injuries.

Movement with a high center of gravity and stiff, unbending knees increases the likelihood of falling. Stiff knees necessitate a sway back which removes pelvic support. Body weight is locked in the chest creating an accident waiting to happen.

A low center of gravity and noticeably bent knees are central to all athletic training. When body weight is centered in the pelvis, the feet become simultaneously heavy and light. One is sure footed and sensitive to holes in the terrain or obstacles in the path. The lower body is full of weighted energy, yet one can walk on onion skin paper without a rip.

It's a tad alarming that in general the elderly are not given the above information by word or workshop. Senior Centers should offer workshops of this nature. Tai Chi classes would be a great idea.

Standard advice for avoiding falls is of a more yang/LB mode such as follows:

- Keep floors and walk ways clear of all clutter.
- Install handrails on stairs and steps.
- Avoid throw rugs.
- Keep a phone in near reach at all times. (That's so that if one doesn't die by fall one can die by cell-phone. Stephen King would agree.)
- Drugs can interfere with balance therefore special care is needed with elderly who are taking prescription drugs.

**Exercises**

Imagine a two foot board tightly secured to the lower back. Sit, stand, reach and move with the board-image making it impossible to bend from the waist. Bend forward from the top of the legs.

Practice walking at various speeds with knees bent and imaginary board at back. Roll through on the feet - heel, ball toe. Don't hit hard on the heels. Move as though a rope, attached to the Tanden, is pulling you forward. This encourages movement from the pelvis instead of leading from the head, neck and shoulders. Initially this may feel strange. Practice will make it natural; it's much easier than dragging the body around by the head, neck and shoulders.

Listen to the sound of the feet hitting the ground surface. A thud sound indicates the entire foot is hitting at once instead of rolling through heel-ball-toe. It is a potentially dangerous, impractical and ungraceful way to move.

Avoid falling into bad habits by observing yourself walking toward a mirror. Is each side of your body a mirror image of the other side? Is one side lower or higher than the other? Is your head in front of the pelvis? Do your arms swing an equal amount and in similar fashion? Is your movement easy and graceful? Do your knees bend with each step?

Hiking mountains is the perfect place to synthesize balancing techniques. Moving down steep inclines is difficult when energy is centered in the chest. When climbing ladders and walking steep rooftops, make sure the legs and feet are moving the body.

*Take a pendulum with you*
*Wherever you go.*
*Resolve your dilemmas*
*The pendulum knows.*

# Developing Intuition

Zen practitioners say the intellect toys with concepts that only intuition can understand. Suzuki, who brought Zen to America, wrote "Intuitionalism requires pointers more than ideas to express itself and these pointers are enigmatic and non-rational. They are shy of intellectual interpretations.......They are like flashes of lightning. While your eyes blink, they are gone."

We reel with indecision. The anxiety attack begins. What to do? What to do? Call on intuition. It's always there, waiting for the opportunity to guide a situation to a positive solution. Intuition is the immediate knowing of a truth without employing the process of reason. It's a flash that compels an idea, concept, action or *knowing* that hasn't been determined by the voice of reason.

Intuition comes in many forms, the most common being inner-voice, feeling and visions. An *inner-voice* intuition probably saved my life. It was late at night as I walked slowly up a very long flight of subway stairs. Midway up, my inner-voice commanded, "Move it! Fly! Faster!" I ran up the stairs, grabbed the railing and jumped steps to clear the area. At which moment a large tree in a pot crashed onto the stairs from hundreds of feet above.

*Feeling* intuition is somewhat different. A friend and I went to a music rehearsal at the apartment of a guitarist we didn't know. A few minutes into the rehearsal the guitarist left the room and I urged my friend, "Let's get out of here now." "Why," he asked. "I don't know why, it's just a very strong feeling." My friend stayed and I left to find a different guitarist.

Several evenings later, we were driving to the performance venue at the St. Regis when the original guitarist said "Jane, I have everybody else's phone number but I don't have yours; you never know when I might hear of a gig in the future." I said "Sorry, can't tell you." Intuition would not allow me to tell him.

Days later, the guitarist made the front page of the New York Daily News. He was discovered keeping a dead woman's body in an air-conditioned room in his apartment. The body was there on the afternoon of our visit. Before the news hit the stands, he stole my friend's musical instruments and sound system. This way-out story happened back in the '70s so I checked with the friend involved to be sure the details were correct. He concurred.

*Visions* are more individualized and always come in moments of silent reverie. My experiences come in moving-pictures superimposed over reality. Example: I was looking out a window overlooking the Empire State building. All of a sudden high walls of mud rolled across the sky toward me blocking out the skyscrapers in the background. Several days later I heard the exact experience described on TV news in reference to a Mexican earthquake.

Everyone is born with intuition. The ability becomes dormant when lifestyles are not compatible with its generation. Try the techniques for releasing intuitive power and discover which approach works best for you. If you fail with first attempts, don't give up. Your ability will improve with experience, concentration, relaxation and a request for necessary information.

## Techniques

- Ask a brief, clearly worded question regarding the input needed. Clear your mind of opinion and random thought at the moment of asking the question. Sustain the empty state.
- Repeat the question 3 or 4 times, using the same wording at each repetition. See the subject clearly in the mind's eye. An overall feeling may accompany the initial phrasing of the question; the feeling is part of the intuitional insight. You'll know when it happens.
- The answer comes when needed. When the question concerns an immediate situation, the intuition often comes within minutes of the question. On other occasions the answer may occur hours or days later. It pops-up when least expected. Practice makes perfect and reveals modified techniques suited for the individual and situation.
- Visualization is another technique that invites intuitive insight. Let's say you can't choose between two professions. Visualize the details of mastering and living the two professions. Visualize living all the details of achievement in each profession. You'll know what choice to make.

- Trust body action in dangerous situations. For example, one is alone in an isolated country home. Intruders have scaled a fence and entered the porch area. The phone is two rooms away; your gun is in the opposite direction. The subconscious knows what to do. Go with spontaneous action, it will move you along the safest path.

- Meditate. Visual intuition occurs in meditative states when thinking of nothing in particular. In a flash, a picture will superimpose itself over your view. Always stay with the image. Ask questions and discover where it takes you. Don't worry about confusing intuition with paranoia, fear or normal intellect. Intuition is easily recognized. It's a total knowing, without doubt or internal argument.

You may find it fun and interesting to try the pendulum for receiving input from the subconscious mind which is always in touch with the Field. Many readers have probably tried it with varying success. I've found it to be accurate 75% of the time and offer the following input.

Hold the pendulum with one hand and brace with the other hand to assure you are not producing any movement. I put it up to my forehead, with two elbows on the table making a tripod.

**Turn off all electrical devices. They will affect the reading.**

Be in a meditative, balanced state of mind.

The first stage is to determine the yes and no responses to your questions by asking the pendulum to show you the directions of the swings for various answers. A majority of dowsers use a vertical swing for *yes*, a horizontal swing for *no* and an diagonal swing for *uncertain*.

Ask an obvious first question to determine if the proper process is underway. I ask, "Is my name Jane Odin." If it answers "Yes" then I proceed. If the answer is *no* I relax my upper body and move to an objective emotional state. If this doesn't work I wait until later; there is apparently a block to accessing the Field.

Some of the most valuable input from the pendulum has been working with animals when they are sick. It's the middle of the night and I need to decide whether to bring the stricken one to the Vet. I hold the pendulum directly over her and ask a series of questions. Acting on the outcome of the swings has always produced great results.

Determine the validity of the reading by looking at the whole picture – the way the answers relate to each other and the vitality of the pendulum swings. An example follows:

After an injury to my head I refused to go to hospital and consulted the pendulum, first asking "Is my name Jane Odin?" It said yes. Next I asked if the injury was life threatening and got a no. The questions continued:

- Do I need to go to the hospital? NO
- Is the injury serious? YES
- Can I take a hot bath? NO
- Do I need to stay awake with head elevated? YES
- Was dehydration the cause of the fainting? YES

Sometimes the pendulum, displays a very small swing. Not the case here. The pendulum moved with an unusual power, giving me great confidence in the answers and basically saving me the monstrous hospital bill I would have incurred.

The first step for easy access to your individual preference of intuition technique is asking a clearly worded question. This will open the door to your best mode of operation be it telepathy, clairvoyance, dowsing or visualization.

*When you're in your 70's*
*Don't grow old and hazy.*
*Get up off your duff*
*You'll lose it if you're lazy.*

# Keep Moving

"Conclusion – Long-term regular physical activity, including walking, is associated with significantly better cognitive function and less cognitive decline in older women." *Journal American Medical Association*

Great news: we *can* create new neural pathways in the brain well into our eighties and probably beyond. It happens through the process of neurogenesis which is the ability of the brain to grow new neurons. The active ingredient in the growth process is a protein called brain-derived neurotrophic factor (BDNF) which also connects one neuron to another - a result necessary for higher brain function. These are fairly recent findings.

The increased production of BDNF is under the control of a gene activated by voluntary physical exercise. Research with the elderly has shown: physical exercise for 20 minutes a day for 24 weeks improved memory and other cognitive functions such as language/speech and focus.

It's all up to the individual. Not only must one exercise daily, but it must be done in the right spirit. You initiate the exercise and enjoy the work out. Otherwise it won't produce desired results.

In 2001 Dr. Guang Yue, an exercise physiologist at the Cleveland Clinic Foundation in Ohio, made an amazing discovery: *mental images of exercise = effective exercise.* Ten volunteers took part in mental workouts five times a week. They imagined lifting heavy weights with their arms and increased their bicep strength by 13.5 per cent. "Muscles are prompted to move by impulses from nearby motor neurons, and the firing of those nerve fibers depends on the strength of electrical impulses sent by the brain." The gain in strength lasted for three months after they stopped the mental exercise.

If you are not familiar with an exercise regime you might watch an *exercise DVD* appropriate for your physical needs. It will certainly help to know techniques of a work-out experience before creating it mentally. And remember the well know admonition: check with your doctor before initiating a serious exercise program.

Gene D. Cohen MD was a major force in the field of geriatric psychiatry and an expert on what happens in the aging brain. Writing in *The Creative Age: Awakening Human Potential in the Second Half of Life* and *The Mature*

*Mind* he glorifies the actuality of those in their 70s and beyond leading creative, healthy lives.

Changes in the length of dendrites in the hippocampus improve memory formation by allowing greater synapses activity. Creativity is the key to accessing the ongoing developments in the brain. That includes everything from art to creative problem solving. Cohen founded Genco a game company that designs board games for the elderly including Alzheimer's patients. They all work on improving memory function.

Contrary to the belief of the younger generations, the elderly are quite astute and remain productive into their 80s and 90s. Throughout *The Creative Age* Cohen presents an endless array of individuals who contributed major creative work in their late 60s – 80s. In his insightful book he mentions an exhibit at the Corcoran Museum of Art in Washington in which 16 of the 20 artists had started their art after the age of 65. Thirty per cent were over the age of 80.

New studies continually reinforce present knowledge that mental capacities expand throughout old age, showing noticeably greater ability at Bimodal consciousness between age 50 – 70. This means there is greater integraton of the two brains, enriching the creative process which in turn reinforces mental acuity.

There are many examples of the elderly who didn't become decrepit and set in their ways. I knew a 78 year old woman who earned a black belt and Lena Horne looked and sang fantastic in her 80's. I regularly watch 75 year old martial artists on YouTube doing demanding Katas (pre-arranged forms) and staged fighting. Some of the great Sifus continue teaching into their 80s. There are endless examples of people who have vanquished old-age through dedication to creative projects and exercise. Never retire to the rocking chair. Keep moving.

Until the mid '70s the field of gerontology generally viewed old age as a disease. Perhaps this is due to the negative effect generated by Freud and Piaget. Freud believed "old people are no longer educable" and Piaget thought intellectual development began to deteriorate in middle age. Cohen's discoveries encourage new understanding of the aging mind and discourage ideas of the elderly as a disposable society.

One never knows the delightful surprises awaiting the young at heart. Don't rule out any possibilities. A favorite story goes like this. Judy went into a retirement home at 80. She dressed with great flair and always had marvelous stories to share, full of laughter and surprises. She fell in love with a 70 year old man she met at the home. The relationship lasted until her death 6 years later.

It's important to stay physically fit throughout life in order to be prepared for elderly years. I started martial arts training at 43 and it became one of the most important disciplines in my life and continues to be a great passion.

Practice Preventive Medicine. Don't turn well being over to Western Medicine. Research problems on the internet and in healing journals such as the "Townsend Letter – Examiner of Alternative Medicine." Once started your inner guidance will lead toward relevant information.

Prayer is a powerful tool in life and particularly in the healing process. Atheists can pray to the Creative Force. It all works equally well because it is the belief of the one praying that turns the tide of life.

Skies are covered with chemtrails (not contrails) dispersed for all kinds of radical experimentation. The chemtrails contain aluminum for reflective purposes. Aluminum leaches potassium from the body creating a myriad of serious health problems particularly for the elderly. I take one 99mg potassium with its companion magnesium (one 250mg) daily. Magnesium is also a harmless muscle relaxant which I find a great blessing under many circumstances.

Living in an extremely dry climate I have become dehydrated to the point of horrid nausea. At which point I take 2 tablets and the problem is apparently balanced. Before learning this little *technique* I experienced some really uncomfortable times.

Potassium is an extremely powerful mineral; it regulates energy exchange in the body. I usually don't take more than one tablet a day. Read about it and/or consult a doctor of alternative medicine.

Plan diet, vitamins and mineral supplements to accommodate known weakness. For example, a long history of digestive problems begs for a meatless diet, particularly for the elderly. This is because the amino acids needed to digest meat are less available from the pancreas. One doesn't want undigested meat stagnating in the gut for weeks and longer as known to do. And keep moving!

Stay involved with creative projects. As Dr. Cohen writes there are large creative projects and small creative projects. The point is to be seriously plugged into some kind of problem solving, be it a totally new recipe with unfamiliar ingredients or a home improvement project. It doesn't matter what it is as long as it's enjoyable, involves original thinking and encourages problem solving.

**Practices**

- When tired, depressed, feeling aches and pains, it's time to walk, swim, golf, bike, garden, travel, stretch, clean the house. Exercise is imperative.
- Most chronic lower back pain can be alleviated with an elastic back support. Many clients have found relief shortly after tightening the Velcro straps.
- Continue yoga, stretching and Zen diaphragmatic breathing throughout life until the final breath. This includes those hospitalized and in nursing homes.
- Stop couch potato inactivity by removing TV or limiting time watched. There are many ways to exercise while watching the tube.
- Meditation will change your life. It can be practiced anywhere. Give it a try!
- For those who are physically able I recommend *Chi Kung; Way of Power* by Master Lam Kam Chuen. It is full of simple exercises and movements that are beautifully illustrated and simply explained.

*Send your beam*
*Into the future*
*Be amazed at what you see.*

# Personal Radar

In *Tao of Jeet Kune Do* Bruce Lee writes one should be alert to the interchangeability of opposites and not let the mind stop with either of the opposites. "A JKD man should keep his mind always in the state of emptiness so that his freedom in action will never be obstructed."

Bruce Lee teaches one can be prepared for any eventuality by living in a meditative state. *Neutral alertness* allows one to move freely and without fear in all environments. Mental neutrality is alert without emotion or opinion. Physical neutrality is poised and uncommitted, ready to move in any direction at a moment's notice. The integration of mindfulness, centering, balance, posture and diaphragmatic breathing moves toward neutrality. A radar type of perception is the culmination of these techniques.

Think of yourself as a powerful transmission station sending and receiving information over great distances. Believe in this transmission capacity. Ask simple, clearly worded questions. Repeat the question several times with full concentration on the question, such as "Is Joe safe at the playground?" Visualize the child in the playground while repeating the question. A frequency-wave of energy goes to the child and returns with an insight or feeling. Remember those streams of photons radiating from all living matter - this is their realm of action.

Close your eyes and release energy from the body in all directions as in the *radiating light exercise.* You will feel a sense of weightlessness and a sense of taking up more space with the physical body. Maintain wide bands of radiating energy as you project the question. At some point later you will receive a good or bad feeling with accompanying visual and auditory details.

One evening I left my country home in Georgia to travel 20 miles on bad winter roads. I sent out my radar as I was opening fence gates to leave and received a puzzling response: "You will have a scary event happen on the way, stay calm and you will arrive safely." That's exactly what happened. Approaching Potato Creek Bridge I saw lights flashing in the distance and thought this must be the event I was warned about.

Remembering guidance I rolled onto Potato Creek Bridge at 20 miles an hour just in case there was ice which couldn't be seen in the dark. I hit a sheet of ice, spun the car out of control and rammed it into the guard rail before stopping. Perhaps if I had not checked things out as I was leaving, I would have hit the bridge at 60 mph and ended up in the river 150 feet below, like the truck that went over a few minutes before I arrived.

Another Georgia experience comes to mind. I was on a barn roof several hundred feet from my home, where I had left my Chow on the porch on a very long chain. She had just had a bath and needed to dry before running about. Fortunately I thought about her well-being in the midst of work and immediately got the message to get to the house quickly. I got down and raced back to the house to find her hanging by her nails from the porch. She had jumped off the side of the porch and the chain was too short. If I hadn't arrived when I did she would have hung herself. I hope these personal stories will encourage you to develop your radar and practice regularly.

## Test application

For a designated time period, at least a month, take every natural opportunity to test your *telepathy* For example, get together with a friend who shares interest in psychic development. Sit across from each other in a quiet space. The friend will concentrate on a very specific image and you will *tune in* the image projected.

I did a trial test with the following results. As my friend projected an image, my mind raced with possibilities. I calmed the clutter by repeating: *release, breathe, release, breathe.* As this process was initiated I closed my eyes.

A string of answers popped through my head; I asked myself silently, "Is that it?" "No" was the answer. Then all of a sudden a bright colored picture appeared on the inner screen of my closed eyes. It was a line of strange birds flapping their wings back and forth, instead of up and down, in perfect unison. "Birds. I see a horizontal line of birds flying with wings flapping in a very unusual manner." My amazed friend replied, "Yes, I was projecting a bird scene from the Hitchcock film, The Birds."

Try silent communication with your pet. Choose a time when pet is in relaxed mode and repeat a silent, simple command such as *come* or *lie down.* Visualize the animal executing the command. You may be amazed at the results. The same process holds true for communing with wildlife.

It helps to have an affinity with the creature to be summoned. Create your meditation and image the creature, say a Raven. See the Raven in your mind's eye. Think of qualities of the Raven and call out loud, "RAVEN."

Remote viewing is another form of human radar that has been popularized recently. Guidance for remote viewing always stresses the need to totally empty the mind and establish slow, Zen breathing. Close your eyes and await the dark screen that appears when the mind is emptied.

Next one learns the difference between images created by imagination and remote-viewing images. Remote target images are usually fuzzy, hazy shapes and colors. If you can easily identify the object then it's probably imagination. David Morehouse is the leading teacher of remote viewing – conducting workshops entitled The Explorer Group.

As with all endeavors – success demands belief. Believe you're capable of remote viewing or it won't happen. Belief, relaxation and Zen breathing are the foundation demanded in this process. They are also the focus of **overcoming contraction** section.

We know from an incident revealed by Jimmy Carter that remote viewing is an achievable reality. A Soviet plane went down in Zaire and spy satellites couldn't locate the wreckage. Remote viewers found the wreckage prompting the CIA operations officer to conclude, "It is my considered opinion that this technique – whatever it is – offers definite operational possibilities." *Mind-Reach, Scientists' Look at Psychic Abilities* by Russell Targ and Hal Puthoff considers details of techniques used in this process.

Work at night to lessen the electromagnetic interference from non-stop bombardment of MW frequency, unless you have it pulsing inside your house. In which case, I would be surprised to hear of your success with personal radar.

*You are a radiant being
With eyes full of seeing
All is one.*

# Charisma

"This little light of mine I'm going to let it shine. This little light of mine, I'm going to let it shine. This little light of mine, I'm going to let it shine. Let it shine, let it shine, let it shine." *Harry Dixon Loes*

Marilyn Monroe, wearing a scarf over her head, walked down the street with a friend and passers-by didn't recognize her. Her friend was surprised by her unanimity until Marilyn explained she had her light turned off. "Watch what happens when I turn on my light." Marilyn did nothing apparent to change herself externally, yet suddenly pedestrians were running toward her calling out, "Marilyn, Marilyn."

Christ, Saints and mystics are often pictured with a halo, suggesting the ability to radiate light. Performers are called stars because they shine with charisma. In Kubrick's film, *The Shining*, the child protagonist has the ability to see *shining* from the Field.

I learned the *radiating light* practice from the Sufi mystic Pir Vilayat at one of his glorious retreats in upstate NY. It was my first experience with meditation and the practice had a sublimely powerful effect which I later shared with my NYU students. They encountered several problems the first time they did the practice: inability to sit still, high chest breathing and repetitious swallowing. Overcoming these obstacles afforded the perfect arena for integrating diaphragmatic breathing, and centering in the Hara.

After our first success with the practice we sat in a circle discussing their experiences which included seeing auras and shadows surrounding fellow students. They saw some radiant beings and some who were drawing light into their darkness. It was most interesting and one student made a memorable contribution saying, "It's incredible, but what do you do with it at the supermarket?" I replied, "This isn't supermarket mentality."

Now – many years later - I see that it is supermarket mentality because without the abiltiy to *see* energy it's hard to determine the real from the false at any level. Looking in wide focus reveals otherwise hidden details which you might want to know about, particularly in the fresh-produce departments.

I recall going into a ghetto supermarket and seeing piles of fruit with no light emanation. There was a darkness hovering over the entire presentation. Needless to say, I decided to forgo the savings. Details of this nature are detected in wide-focus.

### Radiating Light

Take a meditation posture and use meditation techniques with eyes closed. Total stillness is required as you imagine a golf ball sized light two inches below the navel and midway between the front and back of the body. See the ball of light with the mind's eye.

Breathe into the center of the ball of light. Visualize the light expanding with each breath. The expansion continues until there's a sense of light filling the entire body and breaking through the skin surface in thousands of pencil-point thin rays. Visualize the rays moving out from the body.

Ignore superficial pain such as a foot going to sleep or a cramp in your side. Relax the area of discomfort by breathing into the area and feeling it expand with each breath. The key to success is remaining still throughout the exercise.

Run an inner monologue suggesting what is to occur. For example: *I feel a ball of light expanding with each breath. I feel the light expanding throughout my body. The light is radiating through my skin pores, creating millions of light rays.* Open the eyes and look around. The environment will look quite different. Sensitivity to light and shadow is greatly enhanced. The eyes are in wide-focus and perception is heightened.

Walk around maintaining the experience. When it begins to fade, focus on the light and use wide-focus vision. Practice until you can turn on *the light* at will.

Initially the exercise takes 30+ minutes. You don't have to achieve the ultimate to receive benefits. You'll experience direct contact with your energy flow. For example, if you shift into high chest breathing, you'll feel energy moving up toward your neck as soon as it happens.

Try the following experiment when mixing with others at social gatherings, or in a performance situation. Arrive at the destination and mingle without doing the *radiating light* exercise. After a period of time go out for a while and then return doing the *radiating light.* Check out the reaction from folks. Is it any different? You will see a large difference in the surroundings and the effect you have on others.

In the course of directing theatre and conducting workshops for actors it was evident that running a very real, moment to moment inner monologue greatly increased personal charisma. It created energy noticeable to all viewers. When one has something going on internally it is communicated in silence as clearly as when audibly expressed. This was clearly illustrated when an Off B'way play was in trouble at the time of dress rehearsals.

The lead actor called me in to assist in making his role more interesting. This was a little tricky since he was playing a mute creature from outer space. He wore a cumbersome costume and expressed little behavior so our options were restricted. I asked what he was thinking on stage and he said "basically nothing." I suggested doing a radiating light monologue and it worked; the director was thrilled with his *new energy*.

Imagine the ball of light at the level of the Tanden as you go about daily activities. It encourages one to live and move from the Hara, which is characterized in the tumbler-doll with a round, lead weighted belly which always brings the doll back to its original position whenever knocked over. The Japanese ideal of beauty is a being well grounded in the Hara/Tanden. (As often mentioned – the Tanden is located within the Hara, two inches below the navel.)

It's interesting to closely observe people and determine the source of their charisma. Imitate movement, including mannerisms and how they walk. Analyze every aspect of style of dress and vocal expression. Are there commonalities among the most charismatic?

Radiating light in the Hara activates the area, overcoming entrenchment in the upper chest. The body center is carried in one place or the other; we never want it to be in the upper chest. It will interfere with the flow of energy.

Pir Vilayat said that to become a body of light one should be aware of burning with a bright flame that has the feeling of being an incandescent, transparent crystal. In his magnificent book *Toward the One* he has much to say about *light practices* which were primary to his teaching. Because this 673 page volume is out of print I include the following quote and suggested practices.

"One has the feeling of being porous as a magnetic field, crystalline or translucent as an aura. The body of light extends, there's no skin on it, no edges, no frontier. It exudes rays; it radiates….The aim of these practices with light is to envision oneself as a pure light, part of the world's light, by becoming sensitive to one's natural luminosity, to discover within oneself a sense of transparency within the spaces between the atoms or cells of the body Become like a crystal, crystal clear, totally receptive to the passage of light….Instead of visualizing translucent angels, discover your own ability to let light pass through your physical body. Become non-solid; let the breeze blow through you, the light pass through you. Become pure spirit....Discover yourself as a being of light, not as an aura but as a pure luminous consciousness which lights up all things as it turns toward them."

Use Pir's words as a guide for composing a personal inner monologue to increase charisma and raise personal frequency. For example: *I am a radiant being of light glowing with love. Light is moving through every fiber of my being as I soar across the universe radiating a shimmering glow to the north, south, east and west.*

*Tune up your radar*
*Know which way to go*
*Life is full of surprises*
*Stay alert in Kokomo*

# Be Prepared

Daydreaming and forgetfulness at the wrong time and place can create inconvenience, loss or great misfortune. Live in the moment. Focus on the task at hand while maintaining a keen awareness of the environment. Always include inner guidance, particularly when it advises against usual habits of behavior such as the example that follows.

I was attending a Halloween Masquerade Party with two friends. We were all having a great time. Suddenly I *got the message* and told my friends we needed to go. They agreed. I walked to the car and waited but they didn't appear. I waited. This happened twice, as my urgency escalated. My third return, I stood at the terrace doors and screamed their names, over the live band and hundreds of folks having a blast. "We are going now!"

As we drove to Julie's house I explained my overwhelming alarm to get there quick as possible and I didn't know why. We arrived and Julie insisted we come inside and visit for a few minutes. While inside she started talking about her husband and I whispered "No, he is listening" and pointed quietly toward the wall of the next room. Shortly thereafter I left with my other friend.

The following morning Julie called to tell me that if she had arrived a moment later, her husband may have raped her gorgeous, teenage daughter. He had crawled into bed with her and was fondling her at the very moment we drove into the driveway.

What does this story have to do with being prepared? Why did I receive *the message* to leave immediately? Being a non-drinker, I was stone sober and although involved in the evening's activities, I took a moment to formulate the question: "Is there something happening I need to know?" If the question isn't asked the answer may not arrive.

Take guidance with you where ever you go and stay in tune by asking pertinent questions such as "Is there anything I need to know?" And of course, too much alcohol transports one into the never-never land of forgetfulness. That is the purpose of alcohol isn't it?

According to the news media, people continue making careless mistakes that cost lives. So many tragedies can be averted by following common sense.

## Rules of Preparedness

Most of the following apply to city dwellers and one may think them quite obvious. Problem is people keep making the same errors of judgment. So here goes.

- Keep keys easily accessible. Have one place to keep them. Mark or organize keys to avoid fumbling and always keep them in the same place.
- Lock the door immediately upon entering your city home. Never leave the door ajar while rushing to answer the phone or check mail. Someone could be watching and enter immediately behind you. I know of two tragedies that resulted from this exact scenario.
- Never open the door to a total stranger, even when the stranger is in uniform and has identification. If a police officer is there, call the precinct to confirm his identity. This also applies to highway pull-overs. My mother possibly saved her life by ignoring a police car trailing her with lights flashing and driving to the precinct, at which point the phony cop disappeared.
- When entering a city building, scan the area around the entrance to assure no suspicious types are awaiting the unaware person.
- Park on lit streets and in supervised parking lots. Avoid dark, isolated areas.
- Don't wear expensive jewelry on subways or in dubious neighborhoods.
- Gun owners should attend marksman classes or practice under skilled supervision. Keep gun loaded and in accessible place **out** of the reach of children. If you are afraid to use a gun, don't.
- Go to a public place to seek road directions. Don't ask a total stranger standing on the side of the street.
- When threatened by an aggressor, act very crazy. It works.
- Act on intuition.
- Never flag down a stranger from the side of the road, or go to the home of a stranger for recreational purposes. May sound a little strict but too many stories of unfortunate occurrences develop from situations of this nature.

I live next to Kit Carson National Forest. There have been several fires in the forest which prompted me to put important papers in a safety deposit box and to maintain a variety of large travel bags and super large plastic bags filled with clothes ready to go in the time of an emergency. Also the area around the house is cleared sufficiently to create a fire break.

In winter, when ice and snow abound, I carry a patch of hay in the SUV to enable departure from the forest or wherever. It has saved me several times.

The adage "there but for the grace of God go I" always had a special meaning: if it can happen to others it could happen to me. I won't invite problems with negativity but I will be prepared.

*Bet you don't know
What's in your burger.
Are you still eating
Lots of GMOs?*

# Eat At Great Risk

"Abstaining from meat and poultry is one option, which will lower risk of heart disease, cancer and other diseases....Center of Disease Control reports an estimated 6.5 million cases of bacterial food poisoning each year, with 9000 deaths. Poisoning from salmonella, campylobacter, lister and E coli are all on the rise." *Workbook*, Southwest Research and Information Center

As a teenager I discovered my favorite writers and artists were vegetarians. Da Vinci, Thoreau, Shaw, Tolstoy, Russell are just a few. My hero, Tolstoy was transformed by cutting meat from his diet. His appearance, philosophy of life, politics, life style and writing revealed a radical change in consciousness. The change is well documented in the biography *Tolstoy-A Life of My Father* by Alexandra Tolstoy, 1953.

One of my favorite Tolstoy stories tells of the Empress coming to his country home to discuss her displeasure with his social work. At the first meal she complained about the absence of meat. At the next meal a chicken was tied to her chair with a note suggesting if she wants to eat it, kill it herself.

I stopped eating meat 50 years ago. I couldn't face the health threat and philosophical ramifications. Dad raised cattle. I read all the related journals including the ever available "Livestock Breeder Journal" which advocated 19 synthetic growth stimulants. European countries go through reoccurring periods of banning US beef because of added chemicals and nitrates.

This became popular knowledge in the late '70s when Walter Cronkite announced the danger to women who eat meat. He cited high levels of cancer causing hormones and the use of sodium nitrate to preserve meat and keep it bright red. Nothing has changed. Sodium nitrate is a known carcinogen widely used today in meat for both human and pet food.

Joe Pearce (*Crack in the Cosmic Egg*) writes on another aspect of the meat problem in *Evolution's End*. American meat was fed to a native island population during a famine. The youngest females began menstruation years early; males and females developed breasts. Pearce thinks the hormones and other chemicals in meat are having a powerful effect on children. If you must eat meat, organic, grass fed is the way to go.

The big *chicken expose* was released by the Atlanta-Journal-Constitution on May 26, 1991. Journalists investigated the largest chicken farms and production plants in the US and revealed unbelievable conditions: filthy farms, filthy mega-production companies, diseased birds, maggots in most chicken-parts-buckets and infrequent inspections. The expose resulted in the resignation of the FDA director. Nothing has changed; see the Internet for videos of current conditions.

We all know that advisories regarding chicken are strong and detailed. Juice from the uncooked fowl must not be ingested. Yet I attended a barbecue where the host placed half-cooked pieces of chicken on a plate spotted with fresh, uncooked chicken blood and became irate when it was quietly pointed out to him.

Bacteria in meat are easily transmitted to everything the meat touches. If a head of lettuce is cut on a wooden board where chicken has been diced, you could die from the salad. So give some thought to restaurants frequented.

Hot dogs, chicken parts, canned meat, hamburgers and bacon are known to have high levels of nitrosamines, a fast acting carcinogen that produces many types of cancer. Nitrosamines are found in cigarette smoke, beer, meat cheese, bacon. Smoking and drinking alcohol simultaneously is nitrosamine intensive.

GMOs are another food source that should be avoided. Why are Americans so totally unconcerned about GMOs? There has been little if any consumer pressure to label the Franken-foods. Most people continue to eat the stuff with no question while others spend big bucks for hopefully organically grown produce.

The animal kingdom can distinguish between GM food and natural. Stories from the farm are easily available on the internet. One farmer is quoted as saying, "If you want your cattle to go off their feed, just switch them out to GMO silage." Raccoons, mice, deer, hogs and donkeys are known to avoid GMO when given the opportunity. They can immediately tell the difference while most humans don't notice a thing.

Read the labels on all sweet things. If it lists corn syrup then it's GM. It's hard to find a candy bar or so called organic, commercial sweet without it. And yet, the 2009 issue of International Journal of Biological Sciences published a study showing rats fed GM corn developed serious kidney and liver problems. GM corn is still approved for general use.

According to a 2011 report *Genetic Engineering in Fruit Crops for Sustained Productivity*, the following fruits have been successfully transformed: apple, pear, apricot, cherry, tamarillo, mango, papaya and citrus fruits. The report mentions each fruit with a long succession of genes used for the modification listed beside each one. The citrus includes polyethylene glycol known as PEG.

In an effort to save a few dollars I bought a small bag of tangerines at a large supermarket. I noticed several labels on the outside of the bag but without glasses I couldn't read. Later I bit into a tangerine and it tasted like oil. I couldn't believe it – read the labels and discovered that 4 separate petrochemicals had been injected into the fruit to preserve and beautify. I knew something was wrong before the purchase – my intuition kept saying: *they look too perfect to be real*.

Corn, soybeans (tofu) and canola oil have been made less vulnerable to pesticides allowing them to be sprayed with more weed-killer, particularly Roundup, without killing the plants. GM alfalfa seeds are Roundup resistant; cattle on alfalfa fields are ingesting Roundup along with the genetic chaos by Monsanto. It was permitted by the Obama administration in 2010 with the Monsanto Technology Use Agreement which reads: "*Both the MTSA or IVUA prohibit all forms of commercial seed harvest on the stand. Every alfalfa farmer producing seed of Genuity Roundup Ready alfalfa (GRRA) must possess an additional, separate and distinct seed farmer contract to produce GRRA alfalfa seed. GRRA alfalfa seed may not be planted outside of the United States or for the production of seed or sprouts.*"

This Use-Agreement means if you eat inorganic alfalfa sprouts you may be eating Franken-food laden with residue Roundup. Read Roundup 'instructions' and you may be alarmed. Expense and hidden poisons are good reasons to invest in a veggie garden or veggie co-op. If we are what we eat then quality food is one of our largest assets.

In 2009 the American Academy of Environmental Medicine warned the public to avoid GM foods. They listed the following as possible health risks: infertility, accelerated aging, diabetes, weakened immune system and unusual mutations of internal organs, particularly the gastrointestinal system.

Way back in the 1990s the FDA warned GM foods might create allergies, gene transfer to gut bacteria and new diseases. That's not hard to understand: GM products are engineered to produce a built in pesticide in every cell, which splits open the stomach of insect invaders and kills them.

The most hideous action of GM crops is the communication between the bacterial genes and the immune system. The gene molecules vibrate a frequency signal that prompts the immune system to create inflammation in attempt to kill the invader. Inflammation is a common health issue and often goes unrecognized.

Read *Seeds of Deception* by Jeffrey M. Smith. He covers the entire arena and offers some dire predictions for those who consume GMOs. "Eating a corn chip produced from Bt corn might transform our intestinal bacteria into living pesticide factories, possibly for the rest of our lives."

Wouldn't it be wonderful if we lived in a country where critical issues of this nature were brought to the attention of the masses? Instead we are presented with organic gardens on the White House lawn and a redesigned food pyramid inspired by ex-Monsanto officials lounging about in the Obama administration.

*Loose lips sink ships*
*Down to a watery grave*
*Listen for sweet silence*
*Falling on your ears.*

# Listening

"The most important thing is silence. In the silence wisdom speaks, and they whose hearts are open understand her. The brave man is at the mercy of cowards, and the honest man at the mercy of thieves, unless he keeps silence. But if he keeps silence he is safe, because they will fail to understand him; and then he may do them good without their knowing it, which is the source of true humor and contentment." *Om, The Secret of Abhor Valley*, Talbot Mundy

Who was it that said *it's the province of knowledge to speak and the privilege of wisdom to listen*? I heard it often as a child and it made quite an impression along with the WW2 adage "Loose lips sink ships." Through the years I've found it stimulating to do most of the talking, but definitely more profound to listen.

Does ego, fear, or ignorance shape the content of what is heard? Is it easier to listen to strangers than to friends? Do you enjoy activities that need auditory focus such as the radio or is the T.V. always running, barking out endless ads and sickening violence?

What goes on in your head when listening to someone? Do you tune out when you think you know what's going to be said? Do you cut people off, change the subject and start talking yourself? Do you work out your response while listening, missing a few phrases here and there? Are you tuned out in general?

The way words are put together can reveal more than the words chosen. Prepositions, adverbs, conjunctions change meaning. Tone of voice reveals the energy delivered. Listen for motivation. It's enlightening to uncover the root of the impulse.

What do you hear in the woods and the desert? The auditory experience can be as vital and alive as visual input. Listening to a stranger on the phone can be as revealing as seeing the person. The auditory sensitivity of the blind is well known.

The first time Jose Feliciano, blind guitarist/singer, came to my apartment he moved around as though he lived there. He stood for a moment in the entrance room, turned to the left and walked down a hall past three rooms to the bathroom. "Gotta use the john," he said, closing the door behind him. He knew the location of piano, audio-center and kitchen. I asked, "How do you know where everything is?" He replied, "I listen well. I can hear space and time."

John Gray writes in *Men are from Mars; Women are from Venus"* that men and women listen very differently. Women listen for emotional content and provide compassion and empathy, while men listen to objective details in order to provide solutions. Encourage the mode of the opposite sex; women should listen for details and men can try to get a little empathy going.

A neutral mind-set when listening allows for empathy instead of ego amplification such as thinking personal thoughts and planning future agendas. Hearing your own thoughts prevents listening to others. When tuned into the internal dialogue between hemispheres you are not listening.

An interesting 'listening' experience occurred many years ago on a bitter cold evening on a NYC street. I heard a voice coming from somewhere, "Help me; help me" and found a man crouching in an entrance way with his hand outstretched. My date heard a voice calling, "F you, F you" and was alarmed when I went to the rescue. There was quite a difference in our listening realities.

## Exercises

- Listen more and talk less at your next social gathering. No one will notice your behavior as unusual. Think of having enormous ears and finely tuned antennas. Listen to words chosen, attitude, and tone of voice. Is this listening experience different from your usual experience?

- Most people don't listen well. When communicating with children and teenagers, clarification is usually necessary.
  A few well chosen questions will do the job, such as, "Paraphrase what I just said." Don't be surprised when they don't have a clue. Children listen differently. Try content clarification with your mate and close friends. It can improve communication.

- Go to a party in an objective state of mind and listen dispassionately. Objectivity increases ability to read between the lines without reading into the content. Make it a sort of *remember yourself* exercise.

- Close your eyes and listen for extended periods. Choose a safe environment like when a passenger in an auto, plane or relaxing outdoors etc. Think of other ways to experience the consciousness of the blind. It is obvious they hear much better than sighted-folks.
- In order to hear someone, listen with respect and try hard to find something worthwhile in what the person is saying. If not they will sense it immediately and radically alter their words, intention and emotional content.
- Fine tune listening by tuning into different instruments and melodies within a classical piece of music. Bach is a good place to start.

No argument can take place unless both parties are participating. Next time someone is railing against you maintain your silence throughout. Say not a single word and discover the outcome. It is difficult to accomplish but indicates beautiful self-control, particularly when accomplished without signs of physical tension.

Meditate on listening. Do prejudices, interpretations, attitudes and lack of focus create ineffective communication? Keep in mind cultural differences and vocabulary can create misunderstanding. Maintain eye contact and if the listener's eyes glaze over ask for clarification. Glazing over is the ultimate sign of tuning out.

Be a deliberate listener by reminding yourself while listening that you want to hear what is being said. Reflect and paraphrase to assure impeccable listening.

Castaneda writes that Don Juan implored him: *use your ears and take some of the stress off your eyes.* We relate to the world around us through the eyes – usually talking about what we see instead of what is heard. Explore life with the ears and speak of what is heard.

We all have experiences of miscommunication whether it's travel directions, speaker's intention's or memory of what has been said. Be sure to note improvements and remember there's a big difference between listening and hearing.

It's difficult to know truth in the news media unless one can listen between the lines. Listening between the lines involves using content as an outline signaling the arenas of possibility. For example the government usually announces forthcoming atrocities with seemingly innocent opinions regarding ongoing events.

Anyone who listened carefully to Bush's first address to the people after assuming office would have known the U.S. war machine would soon occupy the middle-east.

When listening, the mouth is shut and according to many admonitions in the Old Testament, a closed mouth is a great blessing. The following quotes impressed me throughout the years and every time I forgot their significance I paid the price.

- Psalm 39: "I will watch how I behave and not let my tongue lead me into sin. I will keep a muzzle on my mouth as long as the wicked man is near me. I stayed dumb, silent, speechless, though the sight of him thriving made torment increase."

- Ecclesiastes 28: "Make scales and weights for your words and put a door with bolts across your mouth. Take care you take no false step through it, in case you fall prey to him who lies in wait."

- Proverbs 11: "Who scoffs at his neighbor is a fool; the man of discernment holds his tongue....He keeps his life who guards his mouth, he who talks too much is lost....Sweetness of speech makes words the more persuasive."

- Aristotle: "The tree of silence bears the fruit of peace."

- Thomas Carlyle: "Under all speech that is good for anything there lies a silence that is better. Silence is deep as eternity; speech is shallow as Time."

- T.S. Eliot: "Where shall the word be found, where will the word resound? Not here, there is not enough silence."

*Life is a game
Played with the self
There's no way to win or lose it.*

# Psychic Games

In *Games Zen Master Play*, R. H. Blyth writes Zen teaches by engaging one in a game whose only answer is a new level of insight. The more difficult the game the more intent the player becomes to realize the hidden secret. The *answer* can very well be *there is no answer* which implies egoless ability *to let go.* The following games bring opportunity for similar insights and reveal sensitivity to subtle indicators. They're a lot of fun as an approach to life that sharpens perception and keeps one in the moment.

Opinion and judgment limit reception. The mind should be a blank space, an empty bowl, a silent arbor. "Zen is the game of insight, the game of discovering who we are underneath the masks and roles of personality." Zen is the game of being awake and the only answer is a new level of consciousness.

All endeavors of a Zen or psychic nature involve the process of relaxation, breath, meditation and the *empty bowl effect.* It is the way of pulling content out of the Field where memory and prophesy swirl in a sea of eternal becoming.

The empty bowl consciousness allows one to contact new information instead of recycling personal frequencies by attracting more of the same. When filled with opinion, judgments, attitudes, one projects these considerations on the new subject at hand, making insight and discovery a distinct impossibility.

Think of life as a joyful game that encourages a daily renewal of *being* rather than a winning or losing. Every day, opportunities abound for exploring the unknown, unseen and unexpected realities with no purpose other than expanding ones awareness. A primary purpose is to enrich the ability to create the empty mind required for psychic games, whatever form they take.

**Games:**

Try *reading* photos of people you don't know. Purpose is to give detailed information about the subject of the photo to a person who knows the subject. There are many ways to introduce the game idea without appearing too bizarre. I'll leave this to your discretion. Actually, it can be a real fun party game.

The technique is simple. Clear your mind and look at the photo in wide focus. Create *consciousness without an object* and wait quietly. Images and information will pop into your head. If not, ask silent questions such as: "What do you do? How do you feel?" With practice you will give a detailed, accurate account of unknown people and events.

Study unknown people at social gatherings. Confirm your 'reading' by talking with the stranger or checking with a friend who knows the subject. You will be amazed at your innate ability to perceive beyond the material world. It's easy and transforms a boring evening into lots of fun and insight.

Follow the instructions and wait until the mind is flooded with mental pictures and information. People carry their history and character essence in an energy envelope that hovers around the physical body. Although you may not see the aura, you'll become sensitive to its essence and information will flow.

Life is a psychic game calling for our active participation. We join the playing field through an ongoing testing of psychic abilities. For example when going to a new place, imagine what it will look and feel like. Imagine arriving, walking about, experiencing the weather and people on scene. Expect amazing results when imagination and interrogation come together in pursuit of the unknown.

It is also enlightening to look for *hidden* words within words such as the following example. Looking at the word 'character', can you see *Hara-center?*

*Moving to the rhythm,*
*Chase the blues away.*
*Sing and swing the melody,*
*Tap your feet and pray.*

# Dancing for Joy

The ritual expression of many cultures is centered on dance. Native Americans dance, Sufis whirl and Balinese trance dance. Witch Doctors and Shaman dance at the heart of their rituals. The only folks I've known not to dance were Southern Baptists back in the '50s.

Dance gives easy access to the soul's expression. It encourages heart and memory to heal through the expression of unconditional love and dream consciousness. It's an easily accessible, reliable method for unifying body and spirit.

Dancing shakes the blues away and unlocks tight muscles while relaxing tense minds. It's great exercise and always makes us feel good. NYC discos used to be full of professional money-makers, TV news anchors in particular, who went dancing nightly around 1 am for the purpose of winding down. It was a ritual for both CBS and NBC anchors and producers in the late '70s and '80s.

This section is for folks who feel uncomfortable dancing. Men usually fill this category. No man in my life has ever enjoyed dancing. They liked smooching on the dance floor but no movement occurred to an up-tempo tune. The younger generation of males has broken the tradition of not dancing. The big dance films of the late '70s and '80s lead the way. Ask around and you may find many who shun the dance floor.

The following techniques will give confidence to boogie anywhere.

**Techniques**
- Listen to a rhythm tune. Focus on the beat. Most Pop music is in 4/4 time. If you can't find the beat, turn the music off and make your own 4 beat counts, moving a part of the body to each vocalized count.
- Listen to the drums. Walk in time to the drum beat, bending the knees with each step. Keep the rhythmic walking-step going and involve the arms in a large, repeating movement or gesture.

- Move the hips from side to side and front to back in time to the music. Take a deep breath, let out a scream and shake those hips. Body weight should be resting on the feet and in the hips. Irregular breathing encourages top heaviness, making for an uncomfortable feeling and clumsy execution. Think of Elvis and don't be a tightass.
- Allow feelings to express through the movements. Your body is an open canvas for expression of love, joy, anger, fear, apathy. Keep the beats going in the walk and hips. Don't censor movements. As long as you move in time with the music, you are dancing.
- Listen to dynamics of the music. Dynamic means *changing*. The time remains the same throughout most pop-tunes, but the rhythm is changing. Usually the tune moves toward a climax by adding instruments and quickening rhythms. Recognize the changes with your body movements.
- Dance on the downbeat. Upbeat dancers bob upward, away from the floor. It makes one look and feel awkward and has a tendency to stiffen the body and throw the dancer outside the experience. This takes practice. Count out loud: and 1, and 2, and 3, and 4. Bend the knees, moving toward the floor on the numbers and back up on the ands. Watch good dancers.

## Shamanic Dance Design

This dance will fill you with energy and prophetic tendencies. You will experience an energized meditative consciousness. Expect nothing and participate daily.

- Stand with extremely bent knees, arms straight out to the sides with fingers spread and a sense of weight in the hands. Maintain a straight lower back with the head directly over rectum.
- Lift feet, maintaining bent knees, in a rhythmic toe-heel pattern.
- When the left foot is lifted the right leg sinks toward the ground. It looks somewhat like Native American dance movement.
- When accustomed to movements give variety to direction, dynamics and arm positions. Arm is allowed to bend slightly at elbows but the fingers remain open with weighted hands.
- When bending forward and back remember to maintain the straight lower back as discussed in *Posture is the Foundation*, which means bend over from below the hip, where the legs insert into the body.

- Now add mindful breathing to the dance. Regulate steps to a counted breathing pattern. Design it to fit your natural breathing cycle. Determine the number of steps needed to cover your natural inhalation and the natural exhalation. Then inhale for three steps and exhale for 3 or 4 steps – whatever is best for you. Maintain mindful breathing for as long as you can comfortably.
- Try the Sufi whirl, being sure to whirl in a clockwise direction with the right arm stretched out in front of you to use as a spotting hand. As you turn keep the eyes on the hand; at the moment you begin to lose sight of the hand quickly revolve the head around to catch sight of the hand again. All dancers use the same spotting techniques to avoid dizziness.

In today's world of drought one might consider a rain-dance to encourage cloud formation and rainfall. Spin around fast in a clockwise direction while chanting an easy to recite, rhythmical chant of your own making. The spinning and chant should revolve faster and faster. Rain dances are found in many agricultural cultures from ancient Egypt to the 20th century Balkans.

Dancing is very therapeutic when one has a kidney stone at any stage of development. Drink a lot of water and dance about with a strong jumping motion. It's helpful at moving the horror out and sure beats spending thousands at hospital.

*Watch the performing moment*
*Capturing what it sees.*
*Does it look like you?*
*Or is it just like me?*

# Monkey See, Monkey Do

It's well accepted that viewing a film depicting violence has the same effect on the physiology of the viewer as actually experiencing the violence. And imitating behavior is as real as initiating the behavior.

Behavioral Science has known since the mid-forties that imitation is a major source of who we are in terms of personality and character. This is true for all living creatures. We all imitate what we experience around us as infants and beyond.

Media watchers know the powerful effect of television on world events. Trends, style, fads and fashion reflect our need to imitate what we see and hear. It's scary that parents allow images of violence and the general uglies to bombard childhood dreams

I came into the classroom a few minutes before the morning bell to find several fourth-grade students putting on quite a show for their peers. I had observed the exact behavior portrayed on a sit-com the night before. They had the behavior down to perfection and it wasn't a pretty picture. I asked what they were doing and what their dialogue meant. They didn't have a clue but their behavior was confident and fully executed.

The tendency to imitate grows stronger with age. In the course of teaching music and performance to children I've observed incredible transformations at around thirteen years of age. Children with delightful imaginations and original personal style begin to copy the dress code, communication skills and general manner of their peers. Those who avoided the *clone-effect* came from strong, loving homes with parents supporting the child's vision of life.

The *clone effect* was dramatically illustrated one day while exiting the supermarket as the lunch bell rang at the local high school. Across the street came approximately 30 students – all dressed in black. At first I thought it was some kind of performance event but as I sat in my car watching I realized they were friends dropping by the market for a bite of lunch.

Dressing all in black was just one aspect of this event. Viewing in wide focus I saw a dance performance in that when one student made large physical gestures the pose would ripple across the crowd. The same was true with vocal expression. It was indeed an undulating clone event which emphasized the desire of teenagers to imitate what they see and hear around them.

Recalling my childhood –before the time of TV – the clone effect was not so prominent. I recall friends doing their own thing, in fact going to extremes to be style-setters and not followers. We never moved in huge groups and took great pride in our originalities. I don't recall ever hearing or using the phrase – *everybody's doing it*.

Under the influence of TV, originality is becoming more and more a thing of the past. How can a toddler experience the wonder of imaginary friends and magical moments with a noise box blaring throughout their waking hours? Even my dogs get up and leave the room when TV is turned on. And now days the screens look like a drive-in movie – those HD, thin screened monsters dominate the family room and can be heard throughout the house making thought and intimacy an impossibility.

One of the latest trends is noticeably sexy clothes for 8 year old children. Now where did that idea came from? Certainly not from the local primary school. Judging from current programming on the tube, fashion designers knew it would go over big with the kids because that's what they see adults wearing.

What better way to control the masses – every aspect of one's belief system is being shaped by the manipulation underway. Are we simply regurgitating TV as a major impulse in our life?

**Exercises**

- Keep a record for a week regarding media input, favorite TV programs/films and role models. Become aware of how your inner monologue is influenced by viewing and listening habits. For example – if TV commercials intrude on your meditations it may be time to reduce viewing time.

- Ban violence from TV viewing for a month and discover a more positive outlook on life. Regular viewing of news media can make one afraid to go outside after dark. Turning off the TV creates silence necessary to receive psychic communications.

- Monitor your child's development with care. Keep in touch with all childhood arenas. Every time a child is allowed indiscriminant viewing of violent uglies, they are learning the experiences observed. You might want to place a sign over the kitchen sink and in your workplace: *monkey see monkey do*.

- Encourage children to develop their own style by asking what they like in terms of colors, textures, patterns, hair styles, shoes and so on.
- Analyze how you are influenced by TV and other sources. Determine what comes from marketplace influence and what comes from hyper consciousness. There should be a noticeable difference. Some influences should be blocked outright – such as infomercials – for an endless number of reasons. Having the TV turned on 24/7 as background noise leaves one open to all sorts of negative influences and unusual programming.

*Water has memory*
*I'm happy to say.*
*Keeping us in touch*
*With all our yesterdays.*

# Water's Magical Memory

In 2001 *The Hidden Messages in Water* by Masaru Emoto introduced us to the magical power of water. Over the years Emoto has written several books filled with remarkable photos of water crystals under various influences such as music, printed and spoken emotions, microwave frequency, TV and so forth. Not only is water transformed by all it contacts, it remembers the contact; water has memory.

At the Aerospace Institute in Stuttgart water changed its' signature according to the touch of the processer. Water was taken from the same source and given to each processer to create a series of drops in a tray format. Unintentionally, each processer imprinted a unique signature on their batch of water drops. The images of each individual processor were quite different from each other while the images of an individual processer were all similar.

The Aerospace Institute also found water subjected to various flowers produced images totally different in every possible way from each other. Each flower had its own signature. I wonder the outcome of water under the influences of a serial killer and saintly being. It would make an interesting comparison.

One of the most powerful indications of water memory is found in Homoeopathy where the more a medicine is diluted the more powerful it becomes. While Jacques Benveniste MD was the director of a lab doing classical research on allergies, a colleague asked to run a homeopathic dilution of a known effective antiserum. The serum was diluted in the traditional homeopathic manner and then added to blood samples. Surprise! Surprise! There were as many cells degranulated by the homeopathic dilution as by the full strength allergen.

The lab did 3 years research on the homeopathic antiserum and found dilutions of 1 billion x 1 billion x 1billion as effective as the original - confirming water memorized the molecule it had seen at the beginning of the dilution process. Water has memory.

I spoke with MDs and Homeopaths regarding the idea of using the Homeopathic approach to pharmacology; the MDs said they knew nothing about Homeopathy and Homeopaths said they knew nothing about pharmacology so it looks like we need to do our own research wherever possible.

Since we are 75% water, the nature of this wondrous element is central to all communication both internal and external. Thoughts and spoken words immediately imprint our water nature making it possible to guide one's consciousness toward intended destinations.

Run an inner monologue praising water when drinking the numerous ounces required every day. Prayer before meals is a must do. I speak of prayer unconnected to religion or a deity such as: *May this food be filled with love, joy and good health and create the healing of my entire being. May this great blessing radiate forth across the universe leaving joyous hearts in its' glow.*

My favorite is a Sufi prayer taught by Pir Vilayat: "Toward the One, The perfection of Love, Harmony and Beauty, The only being, united with all the illuminated souls, who form the embodiment of the Master, the spirit of guidance."

Or simply recite a litany of words before each meal such as love, gratitude, joy, hope and wealth. The words recited direct our 75% water toward a higher consciousness which is then reflected in the frequency vibed across the universe.

Try putting water in a small glass container with words such as *love & gratitude* written on the bottom. Give it a good listen to Bach or other classical music and place in freezer. After the water freezes, take it out, let it thaw and spray it on yourself, family, animals and around the house. It is said to have a powerful effect by those who have used it.

Visit the internet and search for Masaru Emoto and *memory of water*. There is a wide array of YouTube videos showing ongoing research. You will also find those who say Emoto's work is a hoax for the following reasons: no peer review; no follow up research by other scientists and no reproducible results. Perhaps they are conservatives who find mystical implications beyond their purview.

Regarding peer review, I attended a lecture Emoto gave in Taos with the help of translator. He speaks very little English which might make peer review a process he would not embrace. He is a very simple man with absolutely no guile or projected ego. His work speaks for itself.

Numerous research projects have been conducted regarding the memory and consciousness of water. One is out of Russia entitled "Human Consciousness Influence on Water Structure" by Pyatnitsky and Fonkin which concludes "Although we have no explanation of the phenomenon, the data represented in this paper would seem to indicate some human operators can produce a consciousness-related influence on water structure."

Controversy often occurs in response to new information and discoveries outside the mainstream. Remember the response to news the earth was not flat and did you know the sister of the Wright brothers was forced to give up her teaching position because it was determined the entire family was nuts because the brothers were trying to fly?

The list of scientists and inventors reviled as crackpots is quite lengthy and includes the Wright Bros; Tesla; Pasteur: Ohm; Einstein; Crick & Watson (DNA), Copernicus, Isaac Newton, Columbus and others. The *others* reviled and rebuked would easily fill a page or so.

Whatever one believes regarding memory and consciousness of water – we need to drink a lot of it daily. As one ages water content in the body is reduced by as much as 20% which means one must drink additional quantities in order to avoid dehydration. Divide your weight in half and drink that many ounces daily. Although some say otherwise – that is the general consensus.

You may have heard of *Your Body's Many Cries for Water* by Batmanghelidj, M.D. which includes the histories of many patients cured of pain and disease by drinking quantities of water. The water treatment eliminates pain from heartburn and migraine headaches almost immediately. Other conditions such as hypertension, back pain, arthritis, allergies, colitis and body weight respond over time.

Western medicine is aware of the extreme dangers of dehydration. Whenever admitted to a hospital you are hooked up to an IV water drip almost immediately. Better to stay out of hospital by responding to pain and general discomfort by drinking water, keeping in mind Batmanghelidj's caveat, "Do not over drink thinking you can undo the damage of many months or years of dehydration by excessive intake of water in a few days. You need to drink a normal amount every day – eight to ten 8-ounce glasses – until full hydration of the body is achieved over a longer period of time."

*Twinkling consciousness everywhere,*
*Vibrations of love fill the air,*
*You're here - you're there*
*We are together.*

# Eternal Light

"As I stared at the wondrous sight, filaments of light began to radiate from everything on that prairie. At first it was like the explosion of an infinite number of short fibers, then the fibers became long threadlike strands of luminosity bundled together into beams of vibrating light that reached infinity." *The Power of Silence,* Carlos Castaneda

Anyone interested in the matrix of energy vibrating the life of all things should be thrilled with the Field concept. The Field is both the origin and destiny for all that will be or has ever been and is the context for understanding the destiny of individual consciousness when the body dies.

We are primarily water, made of hydrogen and oxygen atoms comprised of photons, neutrons and electrons held together by gluons. This is a central point. Gluons are a form of photon, travelling at the velocity of light, around 7 million miles an hour. They comprise most of the body so it is not remarkable to say with certainty: we are light creatures.

Fritz-Alfred Popp discovered all living things emit a stream of light which he calls "biophoton emissions." This light is used for communication within the living organism and with the Field. Other scientists have confirmed Popp's findings that living matter uses light for instantaneous global communication.

Biophoton-emissions express the health of an organism; cancer cells and healthy cells of the same type, give off different emissions. The biophoton web of light is now considered an interface to consciousness, memory and essence in the Field.

Envision the body held together and controlled by light energy. The brain and seven Chakras (nerve centers) spark the internal organs with electrical impulses traveling neuro-system pathways. It is these impulses that EEGs, EKGs, biofeedback devices and Kirlian photography read. Electrical frequency determines consciousness and maintains internal physiology. When the electrical impulse fails the heart, the body dies and returns to stardust, but what about consciousness?

Consciousness is composed of information extracted from biophotons and processed by the brain via electromagnetic impulses throughout the nervous system. Information is absorbed by the six senses, creating memories which are the essence of individual consciousness. There are physicists who believe memory is stored in the Field, accessible when needed. You simply plug into what you want.

Individual consciousness comes from light; it is stored in the brain as light and transmitted throughout the body as light. It is unique to each individual because we all absorb different bundles of information and vibrate at different rates.

When one dies, spirit leaves the body and 'lives' forever. Individual consciousness exits the body as a unified field of light and achieves timelessness and immortality; photons are not constrained by any rules of the space-time continuum.

Individual consciousness doesn't break apart into isolated photons careening about space. Scientists are confident photons stick together otherwise we wouldn't be able to see a single light traveling for Aeons from a dead star.

What if the "many mansions "referred to in John 14:2 are stratified worlds, parallel universes, that attract spirit-consciousness according to the vibratory frequency of the light-being? A negative life, full of harmful actions will have a different light-code than a spirit-consciousness radiant with love and blessings for others. We do know likes attract – birds of a feather etc. This is a good reason to raise one's vibratory frequency before leaving the body.

If likes attract in the Field, killers will hang with killers and peace-makers with peace-makers in the parallel universes awaiting us. Sounds like a good reason to cut negativity out of one's life. Or we can go with the roll of the dice and possibly arrive in a universe full of stark realities. Who knows for sure? One is reminded of the film *What Dreams May Come* which concerns the mind's creation of the life after death experience.

Theoretical physicists dream of the universe as a large Swiss cheese with each hole representing a separate bubble universe, each with different physics. Concepts of parallel universes evolved when science discovered photons are both wave and particle and can exist in two places at once. They have been trying ever since to reconcile 3 dimensional realities with the 11 dimensional realities of quantum physics.

Hugh Everett III first conceived of parallel universes in 1957 but the idea is still considered way out by most. That's understandable considering the weird components of quantum physics which make it all possible.

A strange phenomenon is the effect the observer has on a physical system. What one chooses to observe alters what exists. Fred Allan Wolf says this effect can't be explained without the existence of parallel universes. Read it for yourself in his book *Parallel Universes*.

For decades New Age philosophers have revealed connections between photons, consciousness and the material world of daily realities. Castaneda, Wolf, Tart, Targ and Puthoff are known mediators of the seen and unseen and they all suggest techniques for experiencing the other side. Aspects of their techniques have been touched on in these chapters.

For those who can't embrace after-life concepts put forth in Christian, Catholic, Mormon, Muslim and other religions, it is a joy to understand – to some degree at least – what becomes of the soul-energy when it departs the body. Its possible soul-consciousness finds realities according to frequency attraction in the quantum worlds awaiting us. And I doubt we will find a mighty God sitting on a throne, full of preconceived ideas, judgment and vengeance. Those beliefs have been designed to control the masses.

You will notice Buddhism isn't included in the list of religions; it is a formidable spiritual philosophy that teaches practices for overcoming the suffering of humanity and experiencing truth, love, compassion, self-knowledge, unity and joy. Buddhism is the only spiritual philosophy that has dialogued for decades with science regarding the true nature of reality.

The Field suggests that the soul continues to manifest in the material world. Reincarnation appears as part of the natural flow of energy throughout eternity. There are various concepts of reincarnation with the Buddhist version having the closest parallel to the Field concept presented here. Basically Buddhists believe a stream of consciousness (light) links life with life – across many realms of existence. This understanding remains compatible with quantum theory and the existence of parallel universes.

All is one; there is no death, only the dropping away of the physical body and the transition into free-spirit. The destiny of one's evolution determines the placement of consciousness in the Field after death. All is possible. Considering the nature of the Field, photon-exchange and transformations continue throughout eternity. We are here; we are there; we are everywhere. There's no such thing as dying.

*You have the answers*
*To create your dreams.*
*Stay with your truth,*
*Send forth your beam.*

# Techniques of Consciousness Expansion

Consciousness expansion occurs in stages and requires certain conditions as prerequisites for the experience. It's challenging to create a compatible internal environment for maintaining the frequencies necessary for insight and personal transformations.

Even in the best of times, we need release from overwhelming contraction misshaping our destiny and blocking psychic vision. Times are hard for many and call for **relaxation and diaphragmatic breathing** as step one to finding peace of mind, objective awareness and reliable guidance through the ever changing chaos of unknowing.

I must reiterate – relaxation cannot take place without diaphragmatic breathing and diaphragmatic breathing is almost impossible without a certain amount of relaxation. The total release occurring at the moment of inhalation is the key to the process. Without relaxed diaphragmatic breathing the practices that follow will have little success.

The **remember yourself** practice *is* a reliable wake-up call for overcoming sleep-walking tendencies. When *yourself* is not remembered, the event will be forgotten over time. It is the unification of the internal *I* and the *alert observer* that creates and sustains the experience.

The general feeling of self-remembering is similar to being in a new and unexpected place or having a very different or life-threatening experience such as the moment before an auto accident when time slows down and every fiber of one's being is super-aware; one second turns into a lifetime.

Recently, on a hike in the forest, I practiced the remembrance with an inner monologue: *I look, I walk, I see, I feel, I hear.* I stayed with the practice and had a delightful experience of heightened reality. I was surprised with halos of light shimmering off trees and bushes while my body was exceptionally weightless. I forgot the practice several times but quickly returned to it when the magical environment disappeared. The difference was so noticeable it quickly woke me up. I can still see details of the event experienced days after the practice. It is a very useful way of overcoming forgetfulness.

Thich Nhat Hanh's **mindfulness practices** will accomplish the same effect. Buddhist texts and science claim noticeable change in perception with daily practice. *Remember yourself* and *mindfulness* practices engage all the senses, remove attitude and judgment and change brain frequencies of meditating subjects hooked up to EEG tracers.

Tart's *Waking Up* covers many layers and ramifications of remember yourself and other Gurdjieff exercises. Tart is an excellent source for further insight into practices that upgrade the awareness of those who "have been dead for many years – joyless automatons who are controlled by mechanical habits of thought, perception and behavior."

We embrace activities that awaken *the sleeper* throughout the day. **Disciplined restrictions** are forced changes that enhance personal awareness. Think about it. Restricting sweets, carbohydrates, alcohol and favorite activities will continually return one to a place of remembrance in the act of enforcing the restriction. Rising an hour early for a daily meditation will accomplish the same. If nothing else it will bring one face to face with lack of resolve which could be affecting other arenas.

Of late I've encountered students who expect to achieve a skill or develop a talent via osmosis. It's a big trend in the new millennium. Parents! When Tim doesn't practice – it's time to stop the music lessons – nothing will be accomplished.

Another important condition for transformation is **quiet solitude,** that ever fleeting, 'dream' reality so hard to come by. It is a monumental achievement to find several hours a day for reflection, relaxation, exercise, meditation and new practices. Without solitude, change will not be of your own making.

Researching the lives of yogis, philosophers, inventors, poets, writers, painters and creative artists in general, one is struck by how they cherished solitary lives. It is said that cave dwelling Rishis' created Yoga hundreds of years before Christ went into the desert in search of solitude and enlightenment.

Most people can't imagine living alone or seeking long periods of solitude without distractions. When solitude is embraced along with meditation, the mind becomes empty. At this point of greatly heightened awareness, one experiences living in the moment and becoming more aware of all aspects of life.

A zeitgeist of corruption, hypocrisy, war and general inhumanity makes it difficult to uphold this next condition. **Avoid negativity!** It should be obvious that focusing on negativity magnifies its' power. Biofeedback technology has proven the relating of painful emotions recreates the identical experience in the subject. Is this why I've never understood psychoanalysis? Perhaps we should keep our own counsel and turn venting into positive outdoor experiences, creative projects and volunteer work.

The expression of negative thoughts can affect every aspect of one's internal biology and particularly the immune system. One needs to cherish thoughts of love, hope, endurance and beauty. Hooking up to positive emotions encourages insight and healing; we are the energy we project and relate to. It resonates in the aura, vibrates in the heart and is attracted by frequency signatures.

**Mudras** are considered finger Yoga and are highlighted in Buddhist and Hindu iconography. They are hand positions used for thousands of years to balance energy and cure disease. Although very mysterious in terms of origin and implication they are known to have positive effects on body, mind and spirit.

One of the best known is the Gyan Mudra with the thumb and index finger gently touching while other fingers are held upright. Many depictions of Christ and Buddha show this mudra which is said to magnify spiritual consciousness and alleviate depression, insomnia and tension. This is the mudra most often used while meditating.

The Apan Vayu Mudra regulates heart attacks when done in the first seconds of the attack. Fold the index finger down to touch the mound of the thumb and keep the little finger erect.

One can immediately feel the Mudra move energy. Put your fingers in the Gyan when retiring at night. Relax with diaphragmatic breathing, maintaining the Gyan in both hands. You will feel energy moving throughout the body in a most unusual manner.

There are many mudras to research and practice according to need and inclination. They are designated for specific health benefits and modes of conscioiusness. You might wish to try creating Mudra *dances,* using only fingers, designed to incorporate the input needed at particular moments in time.

There is an aspect of **meditation practice** not stressed in earlier chapters: the power of sitting absolutely still in the correct posture. One doesn't even have to meditate; just sit. As Durckheim wrote in *The Way of Transformation,* "The practice of keeping the body motionless transforms man's inner being."

Sit on your bottom, *not on your head,* and feel slight pressure against the floor/chair with each inhalation. Without the **release ("Master the Breath")** at the moment of intake, the inner-pressure will escalate until the *pop-your-*

*cork* experience forces movement.

**Prayer** is a powerful force for transformation and one doesn't need to be religious. Work with what you believe because **belief** is the power of the process. When you believe in your process it will work for you.

A prayer is a formal communication with the unseen world be it Christ, Mohammed, Buddha, Krishna, Meher Baba, Wakan Tanka, and all prayers travel into the Field where they are processed according to frequency. After all, everything is light isn't it?

Conversations with spiritual realities need to be consistent in intention and emotionally focused without distraction. Although there is controversy regarding scientific proof of the healing capacity of prayer, Masaru Emoto's water molecules reveal the power of words and energy on water crystals and suggest possibilities for transformation of disease into wellness.

*The True Power of Water* relates wondrous stories of dirty, polluted water being transformed by prayerful meditation. "Indeed the water of the huge reservoir was getting clearer. Before the prayer, there was no reflection on the surface as the water was muddy. Now the trees around were reflected on the surface, forming sharp images."

Keep in mind the power of the personal frequency we broadcast across our environments. Frequency is everything as revealed by Radionics which demonstrates diagnosis and healing can be generated by a frequency machine and transmitted great distances for the benefit of humans, animals, soil and crops. I know someone who works in this field with great success.

Vibrational medicine is based on the knowledge that every living entity has a frequency signature totally unique to the entity. By reading organic samples from the entity – hair, soil etc – the resting frequency can be determined and compared with the problem underway, at which point the radionics machine is tuned to broadcast the healing frequency. Distance is not an issue. Several farms in drought stricken areas have benefited from this quantum science.

**Bimodal Consciousness** sets the stage for expanding consciousness through the synthesis of opposite modes of processing. One of the best ways to practice Bimodal is to **unite passion and objectivity in a sea of moment to moment observation.** That's a very specific objective, and a difficult one to achieve. When accomplished, it's a path of reoccurring bliss.

The RB is the primary seat of psychic consciousness and certainly necessary for moving into unknown dimensions of communication. Theorists are confident of the Field as a *memory holder* which has obvious implications for time travel and remote viewing. If all of history is floating around us, all we need are the techniques and practices to access these realms. In order to see and be, we need a compatible frequency.

Newcomers to expansion-techniques may be LB dominant in which case a focused concentration on expanding RB activities is essential. Find a simple project – such as adding a bit of flamboyance to your style. Paint a self-portrait – to move into the visual/spatial brain and forget words and logic. It's difficult for goal orientated, left dominants to embrace these activities. Just the attempt can turn into a challenging experience.

An impressive example of modes of consciousness occurred on an Oprah Show years ago when an entire audience of men agreed empathy, compassion and emotional expression was not their strength. And above all, they hated having discussions about emotional issues. They all agreed their love was expressed through problem solving and the money they furnished for an upscale life. This perspective indicates extreme LB dominance.

**Wide-focus viewing** is a technique easy to accomplish and revealing to sustain. There is no quicker or more reliable method of seeing into the heart of the matter. Immediately upon switching out of narrow focus one can see energetic connections between living matter. It is the way of viewing light, shadow and auras in human and animal subjects.

Stop talking on the cell-phone while driving. The two don't go together for safe passage. Talking and listening are LB; driving is a RB visual-spatial mode. If you are unaccustomed to bimodal processing, forcing the issue might cause a rude awakening.

Hopefully **moment to moment reality** will become a way of life. It is a best therapy for a worrying mind or a broken heart. It's impossible to be in the past or the future when truly in the moment. Sounds simplistic but not so. When sorrow fills the heart, recite moment to moment realities – just the facts.

Remember the Castaneda quote describing "filaments of light" radiating from everything, like threads of light reaching eternity. His words echo descriptions recorded in near-death experiences and endless metaphysical journals, including Swami Vivekananda's *Raja-Yoga*.

P.H.M. Atwater's wondrous book *Future Memory* contains much on near-death experiences and the effect three such experiences had on her life. In it she briefly mentions **Aka Threads,** a Hawaiian belief that includes a practice of advanced telepathy one may find rewarding to practice.

Basically the Huna belief is compatible with the idea of a perfect union between Quantum theory and morphogenetic fields, which union creates an entanglement that implies a web of light threads connecting all things that have ever been in contact with each other. These connections can be created, strengthened into cords or obliterated at will.

The Hawaiian Huna believe all physical and mental contact with material energy involves the exchange of light threads. Repeated contact creates thicker threads until they become cords of connection. Or – touch a rock and you imprint that rock and vice-versa.

This concept can be utilized to establish contact with anything in the material world and the Field including job opportunities. Meditative awareness of established connections can be used to disconnect from negative relationships.

**Creating Aka Threads**

- Imagine a colored thread of intense light projected from the heart, Hara or Third Eye, arching over to connect with another's power center. You must see the intense light making connection.
- Imagine a colored thread or cord connection with someone at a distance. The thread is created with mental and physical contact. Successful connection should improve telepathic communication.

The act of creating Aka threads is best practiced with people you know. Involve them in your process for several reasons. It allows you both to validate the connection and 2) avoid the possibilities of manipulating others.

Those interested in studying the secrets of the kahuna will want to read *The Secret Science at Work* by Max freedom Long. Long started a research group back in 1948 called Huna Research Associates to investigate the Huna system of beliefs and practices. There is much of interest in Long's books including the following quote.

"To make a precise and clear picture, the kahunas often composed a short prayer describing what was wanted in exact but brief detail. They repeated it three times in succession to make very sure that the picture remained the same and stood out clear and strong. They spoke aloud, as if addressing the High Self, knowing that the Low Self (subconscious) was carrying the picture along the aka cord to the Higher Self."

Eventually relaxation work and expansion practices will become a way of life, both enriching and informing all that you are. People have wide ranging affinities; practices that work best for one may not work as well for others; eventually you will create your own combinations and experience discoveries. If nothing else – it's a fun way to encounter your reality level and envision the unimaginable from time to time.

# Connecting With the Field

*Once I saw a city, hidden out of sight,*
*Protected from the darkness, keeping in its' light.*
*A light of shimmering brilliance so fantastic, so bright*
*And the sounds of joyful music were floating thru the night.*

*A canvas sky was stretched above me and from the center of the eye*
*A film of endless footage was projected on the sky.*
*And I stood with countless others, who were watching, just like me,*
*They stretched on into the distance for as far as I could see.*

*The life of every man was recorded in the eye*
*And projected on the screen, every dream without disguise.*

I wrote the above lyric in the 60s while walking 44 blocks from 86th street to Times Square in Manhattan. The sky opened and the visuals were very intense – as described above. I now realize what I saw was possibly that place known throughout time as heaven, prana, akasha, zeitgeist and the Field. Or perhaps it was a parallel universe – who knows.

I'm confident the experience was prompted by what I was reading at the time: *To Lhasa in Disguise* by McGovern, *Om, The Secret of Abhor Valley* by Mundy, *The Teachings of Don Juan* by Castaneda, and T. Lobsang Rampa's books. They made me aware of extraordinary realities and opened possibilities of seeing worlds within worlds, now considered parallel universes. Once new realities are introduced to the subconscious, they continue to expand, when maintained by constant remembrance. This is certainly true of the Field and makes sense of so many controversial realities.

For example, if the Field did not exist then intuition, telepathy and other psychic awareness could not happen and the work presented here would have less purpose in terms of personal in-sight and communication with the world at large.

Maintaining an open flow with the Field initiates experiences with reliable intuition, telepathy and psychic abilities that allow one *to see* around corners, determine truth, avoid catastrophe and create a healthy, purposeful life. Hopefully the following descriptions will encourage a stronger connection with the Field; **it's helpful to be able to imagine a thing with clarity in order to understand and use it effectively.**

Thoughts and ideas transit the globe at the speed of light. The German philosopher Hegel called the swirling stream of vibrations *zeitgeist,* which translates as *spirit of the age. Zeitgeist* is another name for the oscillating energy fields communicating with each other in never ending space. Although quantum physics supports this concept, the controversy regarding the existence of psychic consciousness continues to rage in the scientific community; strange considering mounting evidence supporting instant communication between and among all realms of *being.*

An exciting example of telepathy within the Field is known as the Baxter Effect, which demonstrates how plants communicate with the world around them – in this case with Clive Baxter, at the time considered the world's leading polygraph machine expert.

Baxter was doing experiments with plants rigged with a galvanic skin response device (GSRD). While measuring the sensitivity of the device he accidently discovered the plant's ability to detect and decode thought; the plant responded on his polygraph machine just like a human being.

When he watered the plant, it immediately responded with a "happy" feedback, long before the water had time to reach the roots. At which point Baxter decided to burn a leaf with a cigarette lighter. His thought caused the plant to immediately respond with a fear response even though he never lit the flame.

Baxter also discovered when the plant was cut it "fainted" producing a flat line on the polygraph machine. This information made headlines in 1966 – along with similar work being done in the Findhorn Garden in Scotland where miraculous gardens were grown in a barren, hostile environment. If plants can respond to telepathic signals it should be obvious that all living creatures have this ability including humans. No doubt about it.

One of the best illustrations of communication within the Field, the 100th Monkey phenomena, supports the reality of telepathy. After a certain number of monkeys learned to wash sand from sweet potatoes in order to eat them, the behavior spread to monkeys on distant islands. Quantum theory would say this is normal communication in the Field. If plants communicate with a polygraph machine why not *monkey telepathy*?

Rhythmic vibrations from an event spread out across the universe at the speed of light. For the most part, they are extremely weak currents, although everything is relative. Way back in the '70s it was known oysters raised together and then separated across the Atlantic, reacted at the exact moment its' partner received an electric shock. Read about this in Bentov's books.

In 1982 Alain Aspect performed an experiment, considered one of the important discoveries of the 20th Century. Aspect discovered photons, under certain circumstances, can instantaneously communicate with each other regardless the distance separating them. It doesn't matter if they are five feet or five billion miles apart.

David Bohm challenged the non-locality of Aspect's discovery saying that yes, photons do recognize each other's presence but because they have no location it is irrelevant to think of them as being separated from each other. In *Wholeness and the Implicate Order* Bohm presents his theory of *reality as* two worlds with a third world as backdrop for the other two which he called the implicate and explicate order.

The explicate order is the world as we know it – tables, chairs, events – in a continuum of time and space. The implicate order is our current world reality without time, space or locality. Both of these realms are enfolded in the Field which contains all that has ever been or will be.

Sounds a bit like a fairy-tale/science fiction reality    - worlds within worlds within all that is, has ever been or will ever be. But Bohm is one of many who speak of this nature of the universe and beyond in similar terms. When one lives with the ramifications of these possibilities – and that's all we can attain to – individual consciousness resonates with a world where *all is one* and information communicates with all that is in the flash of an eye.

Itzhak Bentov's work also supports the 100th Monkey scenario and the idea of parallel realms of *being*. He wrote in *Stalking the Wild Pendulum* "The signal from the movement of our bodies will travel around the world in about one-seventh of a second through the electrostatic field in which we are embedded." It's fairly obvious the 100th Monkey scenario could have occurred; whether it did or not is almost not relevant in terms of possibilities that exist.

Not only does Bentov confirm psychic communication, he also indicates relationships based on frequency transmission and confirms the soul's journey after death. He writes, "Upon the *death* of the physical body, the psyche returns to its realm, finding its proper reality band with which it naturally resonates, depending on its level of evolution."

How do telepathy, parallel universes and psychic transformation occur? The bottom line seems to be the amazing, almost magical photon/ electron that can be both particle and wave depending on circumstance of the moment. It is this ability to be in two places simultaneously that makes expanding consciousness and personal frequency transformation possible.

In *The Secret Oral Teachings in Tibetan Buddhist Sects* we read "There are two theories and both consider the world as movement. One states that the course of this movement is continuous, as the flow of a quiet river seems to us. The other declares that the movement is intermittent and advances by separate flashes of energy which follow each other at such small intervals that these intervals are almost non-existent."

The continuous flow is the wave; the intermittent movement is the particle. The process of transformation is the particle becoming the material world and the wave form becoming parallel universes. This appears to be the connection between seen and unseen worlds. And it is this transformative ability that allows one to raise personal frequency and expand consciousness into vast arenas of communication.

Consciousness is always available for upgrading or downgrading according to the photons integrated into our electrochemical process. As quantum physics says, light turns into matter and matter turns into light. Or as Einstein's Special Theory of Relativity says: energy is mass and mass is energy. Or as Isaac Newton wrote long before Einstein, Schrodinger and Dirac: "Are not gross bodies and light convertible into one another, and may not bodies receive much of their activity from the particles of light which enter their composition? The changing of bodies into light and light into bodies is very conformable to the course of nature, which seems delighted with transmutations?"

Creative people are able to tune into states of consciousness that hook up with inspiration and information in the Field. One may prefer to think of this source as God; that is fine – it doesn't really matter what one calls *it* as long as the connection exists. Our connected consciousness knows how to interact with multiple realities simultaneously.

Everything we do, say and don't do sends encoded currents of energy into the Field. It is most rewarding to develop sensitivity to these encoded currents flying about. A personal example of encoded currents goes like this. I saw a ribbon of light, looking very much like a ticker-tape, cross a large room, moving from Sam toward me with the following info encoded strangely in the band of light, "If you knew what was going on, you'd wipe that smile off your face." It was an unforgettable, momentous experience – because I did know what was "going on" and this unusual event confirmed it.

When one is functioning at the intuitive level, information arrives in sudden chunks of insight. Most often one is not actively thinking about the subject of the insight and the wisdom delivered is outside one's current inner monologue. These are good clues as to the authenticity of the intuition.

We need to distinguish between intuition and imagination. When consciousness *connects* with the Field one's awareness expands to include subtle visuals such as light forms darting about or morphed facial expressions on others. Pictures suddenly appear in the mind's eye or motion pictures scroll on the inner screen. Sometimes you know verbatim what another will say long before you hear it. The same is true for events and experiences in general.

The Field is everywhere; it runs through all things – living and inanimate. Each living essence has a field, like Rupert Sheldrake's morphogenetic fields found in *A New Science of Life* in which Sheldrake claims animals tune into the experience of their predecessors, similar to the 100th Monkey phenomenon. He discusses experiments conducted at Harvard which demonstrate that when a few rats have learned new behavior it transfers easily to rats around the world.

All living creatures communicate within particular frequency ranges. *Birds of a feather flock together* and so do humans of a feather. Experiences are attracted by individual frequencies - w*hat goes around comes around* as one attracts in the groove with one's dominant consciousness. Which means if you don't like where you are now, change your focus, inner monologue, day dreams, routines and general input.

*Remembering yourself* increases contact with intuition, spirit guides and the Field. Sometimes it will prompt an important memory such as happened one morning, as I began a hike. I was already 100 ft or so away from the car when I remembered to ask "is there anything I need to know?' "Lock the car doors" was the reply. I walked back and found the doors were unlocked and yes, valuables were inside.

As mentioned in the Preamble, connecting to the Field is beneficial for the elderly. It will sustain memory, imagination, and creativity and help prepare for the great transition. Arrival at a preconceived destination is not required; curiosity is what sustains or as Lynn McTaggart writes in *The Bond:*" A perpetual fascination with the new appears to be a mainstay of healthy old age." Wherever curiosity takes us is usually a great pursuit to follow.

If indeed, consciousness is light and information is encoded in photons, frequency modification is always available through electrochemical transference. As we think so we call forth from the sea of eternal knowledge. We attract according to familiarity and karmic history (genes) which causes the mind to focus in certain arenas and attract more of the same - unless one determines to call forth new input and thereby transform frequency and essence. Yes, it takes persistent effort and radically new behavior to reinvent oneself and live with open connection to the Field.

# Conclusion

The purpose of writing this book is to share a process that has worked for myself and many students and clients. Embedded in the process is the encouragement to find your path through study and experimentation. Don't take anything at face value and never look to others for the final answer.

It's my deepest hope you will be encouraged to reinforce ever-present wisdom through prayer, mindful practices and meditation, asking guidance – is this good for me? Am I on the right path? How can I humanely serve humanity?

Asking questions directed toward the Field is key for receiving guidance. It is possibly the meaning of *ask and it shall be given unto you*. The various practices put one in contact with reliable guidance and over time one develops an internal switchboard of techniques which can be plugged into for the appropriate mode of consciousness. One becomes more and more familiar with internal worlds and moves toward parallel universes in the Field.

Great change is underway at every level of existence. This should be apparent to everyone, including the living dead. Response to economic and earth changes will define the destiny of who we are as we stick together in a bond of love, compassion and empathy for all creatures, including the precious animal kingdom and the living planet that sustains us.

With greater understanding one loses the fear of death in the material world, particularly since we all face the same conclusion to our 3D reality. Instead, radiate frequencies of love and blessing for all, knowing our vibes encompass all realities and will flow back around to enrich every moment of this life.

Should you find yourself fresh out of love and compassion for others, try passionate pretense; eventually it will turn into the real thing. Temper loving kindness with alert observation and preparedness for any eventuality. This is the way of the 21st Century and so important in today's world of baba sheep and evil bankers.

Keep in mind that **millions of people can't be controlled by a few unless they allow it.** Hopefully, the Wall Street protests spreading across America are the beginning of a universal call to take back our freedoms and create a loving environment for all creatures. The first step is to stop drinking the kool-aid dispensed by the big screen in the living room. The truth is alive within each of us and will manifest as the experienced reality of our time.

## Appendix A

# Beware Plastics

Plastics off-gas organic compounds known to radically interfere with the endocrine system. BPA and phthalates imitate estrogen in both sexes; estrogen is at the root of most cancer and phthalates alter chromosomal DNA (the basic structure of life).

Millions of tons of **estrogen mimickers** are created annually to make some plastics hard (BPA) and others, soft and pliable (phthalates). There's so much BPA and phthalates in air, water and food that **just being alive in today's environment is similar to wearing a sex hormone patch**.

These chemicals amplify the effects of estrogen and produce estrogen dominance in both sexes. In females this dominance encourages breast cancer, stroke, heart disease, hypertension, weight gain and chronic fatigue. In males it may cause hair loss, lowered libido and impotency. Is estrogen dominance the reason for the Viagra craze?

Off-gassing BPA creates chronic toxicity in animals. Over 100 animal studies show results of cancer, obesity, neurotoxicity and breast cancer at low doses. In 2007 a consensus statement by 38 BPA experts concluded average levels in people are above those known to produce harm in animals and there is concern for effects on brain, behaviour, prostate gland and mammary gland in foetuses, infants and children.

Don't look to the FDA to protect us; instead they collaborate with the American Plastics Council and gave the OK to BPA on 9/16/08. On the following day a new study on human subjects published in the Journal of the American Medical Association found BPA strongly linked to type 2 diabetes, heart disease and liver-enzyme problems. But the news had no effect on the feds.

The Sun Online, a British News Journal, ran a story 9/17/08 - "Killer Chemical Lurking in Food" - about research at Peninsula Medical School in Exeter, England that doesn't agree with the FDA. The Brits discovered subjects with high levels of BPA were twice as likely to have diabetes and heart disease.

Phthalates are the most common estrogen mimicking plasticizers and have the unique quality of migrating to the surface of plastic and evaporating/leaching into the environment. This could be a perfect backdrop for a terrifying Steven King horror film.

Phthalate DEHP, a carcinogen found in PVC (polyvinyl chloride) is commonly found in building products, medical devices, PVC toys such as rattles and tethers, shampoo, food packaging, vinyl flooring, hoses, nail polish, hair spray, to name a few. Many phthalates are classified as toxic by EPA's Toxic Release Inventory and researches using human subjects show phthalates create observable DNA damage in the sperm.

The primary route of DEHP exposure is food such as meat, fish and milk. Way back in '92 the International Program on Chemical Safety found the daily intake of the average person to be 2mg. That was 17 years ago - imagine what it is now with fish swimming in seas of plastic & oil and inorganic beef full of additives and who knows what.

The safest plastics for repeated use in food storage are #2, #4 and #5. Plastic #1 (PETE or PET) primarily used for soda bottles, leaches carcinogenic phthalates and should not be reused in any fashion. #7 polycarbonate hard plastic must be avoided. #7 leaches BPA. The Green Guide.com advises removal of deli items from Plastic #3 soon as you get the items home because #3 is made of polyvinyl chloride which leaches dioxin, a carcinogen.

Styrofoam is #6 plastic and associated with central nervous system damage, depression, fatigue and compromised kidney function. Put restaurant orders into safer containers pronto and watch for deli items that have been resting on a bed of Styrofoam.

One of the most accessible sources of BPA is canned foods. Canned soups, pasta and infant formula are found to have BPA levels in the dangerous zone. Some liquid baby formula is packed in containers lined with BPA.

Think of plastics as living entities giving off molecules of life altering chemicals. Plasticizers are found everywhere including the open seas of the Gulf and the North Atlantic, not to mention the blood of most tested subjects. The tragedy of this scenario is the powerful, life-altering effect they can have on the foetus and infant.

Several years ago I removed nasty toxins from my home. My nasties came in the forms of kitchen-plastics, brominated fire retardants (BFRs), vinyl armchair and nylon, stain resistant area carpets. One of the items was with me for decades, causing a friend to remark: "Don't you think you're over-reacting? The damage is done." Funny nobody felt that way when I quit smoking after many years of contaminating myself and the universe.

No, I don't think I over-reacted and neither do my little dogs whose respiratory problems have improved. I even removed the office chair – because it is made of foam and foam off-gases more with age. Why would I go to these extremes? Just knowing the potential of these nightmare chemicals instills abhorrence for everything they inhabit.

Most nylon rugs are treated with super toxic levels of stain-resistance chemicals such as isocyanate, silane and polyurethanes. These are nasty chems known to cause respiratory problems. Yes, nylon is made from petrochemicals, with all that implies.

Watch out for fire resistant hearth-rugs. Brominated fire retardants (BFRs) are unregulated neurotoxins and considered more toxic than PCBs. BFRs are bio accumulative and in minute doses they impair attention, learning, memory and behavior in lab animals. With respiratory systems under attack there's no wonder childhood asthma is the most chronic childhood disease. It's at epidemic levels with one in 13 children wheezing through life. For the bromine atom – it's all in a day's work.

On 8/10/11, the LA Times ran an article entitled "High Levels of Toxic PBDE Found in Pregnant California Women"- a study conducted by UCSF. Ami Zota, lead author of the study said PBDEs are coming from products containing polyurethane foam including cribs, car seats, computers, TVs and carpet padding. Zota advises wet mopping homes, washing hands frequently and avoiding products made from foam.

Wall to wall carpet is one of the more toxic products on the market. A small terrier in Georgia was suffering from extreme, unmanageable allergies and had been furless for over a year. Several months after carpets were removed throughout the house, the fur began to return and now the terrier is fully recovered.

Researchers with detection devices claim the source of most BFR in homes is TV sets. They suggest keeping screen and areas around and under TV very clean, in a manner that doesn't spread dust. Be sure TV is off when cleaning the entire set with a damp cloth. You'll be amazed at the blackness on the cloth.

Unfortunately Americans continue to believe government agencies protect them from industrial chemicals. By now it should be evident nothing could be further from the truth. A must read is "Exposed "where you will learn how the EPA, FDA and American Chamber of Commerce work together with big industry and have failed us big time.

Total avoidance of toxic plasticizers is impossible but there are many things one can do to protect against regular consumption.

- Never microwave plastic. Use Pyrex or other oven safe glass.
- Store food and water in glass containers.
- Remove plastic from the kitchen, nursery and toy-box.
- Look on the bottom of plastic containers and don't use the worse plastics: 1, 3, 6 &7.
- Remove dentures, partials etc at night and whenever possible.

- Plastic wrap made from polyethylene doesn't leach plasticizers, PVC does.
- Backings on new carpets use PVC.
- Indoor plastic materials in vinyl sheet flooring, wall surfaces in bathroom and kitchen may cause respiratory problems. Proper ventilation is important.
- Use glass lenses for eye glasses instead of plastic ones.
- Phthalate DEHP is found in cosmetics, perfume, nail polish, hair spray and is considered a reason for high levels of phthalate in women 20-45.
- Phthalate is found in flea collars. I've had animals all my life and never used a flea collar. In today's world it's good to research every purchase.
- Use glass or ceramic bowls to feed pets.
- Plastics in the dash board and other sources off-gas BPA inside a new car. I can't ride in a new auto without becoming seriously ill.
- Eat a diet high in natural estrogen inhibitors such as broccoli, berries, buckwheat, cabbage, citrus, grapes, onions, melons, squash and green beans.

In the above list I mention becoming ill in a new auto. It happened only once; the experience was so severe I've never ridden in a new auto since. I became what I can only describe as *insanely nauseous*. My body was exploding with nausea as I crawled on hands and knees, back and forth on the side of the highway as my friend looked on in horror. This went on for over 20 minutes. With a little research I learned new dashes give off benzene vapors.

Think about all the ads on TV pushing new, plastic-fandangos for the kitchen. Over and over they show plastic devices being used in the microwave oven. This is an absolute NO!NO! It's bad enough most processed food is wrapped in plastic; we don't need to cook it up for a greater release of toxins.

# Appendix B

# Zapping the Masses

"There is a growing perception that microwave irradiation and exposure to low frequency fields can be involved in a wide range of biological interactions. Some investigators are even beginning to describe similarities between microwave irradiation and drugs regarding their effects on biological systems." *Bioeffects of Selected Non-lethal Weapons*

We know the government is aware of MW frequency hazards: the declassified US Army document *Bioeffects* describes folks 'cooked-up' to create a myriad of effects such as induced fevers, voices in the head, nausea and prolonged hyper-thermia. This important document is easily available on the internet.

The document discusses the use of high frequency millimetre waves at 95 GHz to create "micro-wave-hearing", a silent communication system which involves putting sound and words in someone's head. (It also causes thermoelastic expansion of the brain.) So should you start hearing things it doesn't necessarily mean you have developed schizoid tendencies. The document reads as follows regarding *silent communication*.

"This technology requires no extrapolation to estimate its usefulness. Microwave energy can be applied at a distance, and the appropriate technology can be adapted from existing radar units. Aiming devices likewise are available but for special circumstances which require extreme specificity, there may be a need for additional development. Extreme directional specificity would be required to transmit a message to a single hostage surrounded by his captors. Signals can be transmitted long distances (hundreds of meters) using current technology. Longer distances and more sophisticated signal types will require more bulky equipment, but it seems possible to transmit some of the signals at closer ranges using man-portable equipment."

Risk of Brain Tumors from Wireless Phone Use, analysis of multiple studies on cell phone users, published in 2010 Journal of Computer Assisted Tomography concluded "that the current standard of exposure to microwave during mobile phone use is not safe for long-term exposure and needs to be revised." This analysis was responsible for the warning: *text more, use cell phones less*; they may be dangerous for your health.

The Russians were aware of these dangers back in the '50s when they beamed minus 2.4 frequencies MW at the American Embassy. This is a much lower frequency than current cell phone standards in the U.S.

Clinical analysis by numerous scientists found and detailed the following effect of the 1953 irradiation: chromosomal changes, haematological changes, brain tumours, increased cancer, neurological & cardiac disease. *http://www.emfacts*

58 years later, the Russian National Committee on Non-Ionizing Radiation Protection says persons under 18 years should not use cell phones. Children experience disruption of memory, decline in attention, diminished learning, sleep problems and increased irritability. Russia is one of a few countries to consider the non-thermal effects of RF radiation.

In '92 the Cellular Telecommunication Industry Association (CTIA) asked Dr. George Carlo to direct a $25 million research and surveillance program to assure cell phones are safe. When research produced evidence to the contrary the CTIA turned against Carlo, threatened his career and refused to issue appropriate warnings to the public. All of this info is documented in his 2001 book *Cell Phones, Invisible Hazards in the Wireless Age.*

Dr. Carlo recommends the following for dedicated cell phone users:

- Keep the antenna away from the body by using a headset, earpiece or speaker phone. (This does not include Bluetooth Technology earpieces.)
- Be sure the antenna is fully extended during phone use to avoid radiation emitted from the entire phone and encompassing the entire head. (Now days the antenna is embedded in the phone making the entire phone the antenna.)
- When signal strength is low, don't use the phone. "The lower the signal strength, the harder the instrument has to work to carry the call and the greater the radiation that is emitted from the antenna."
- Don't sleep with phone near bed in the ON position.
- The greatest amount of radiation is emitted during dialing and ringing. Keep the phone away from the body.
- Use cell-phones only for emergency situations.
- Children under the age of 10 shouldn't use wireless devices of any kind.

The Army's *Bioeffects* document was written in '98. Imagine the advancements in microwave technologies in the past 13 years? They can regulate frequency rates of most microwave systems remotely which could transform a DAS grid system into an experimental containment arena. Possibilities boggle the mind as revealed in the *Bioeffects* document: "A variety of innovative uses of EM energy for human applications are being explored. The non-lethal application would embody a highly sophisticated microwave assembly that can be used to project microwaves in order to provide a controlled heating of persons. This controlled heating will raise the core temperature of the individuals to predetermined level to mimic a high fever with the intent of gaining a psychological/capability edge on the enemy, while not inflicting deadly force."

And for those who will ask why the government would allow such a nightmare to unfold I am reminded of a favourite childhood story. Remember the scorpion who asked for a ride across the river on the turtle's back? Initially the turtle refused saying the nasty insect would kill him with a deadly sting. But the scorpion said "Oh no, because I too would drown." "Hummm, that makes sense, climb aboard." Half way across the river the scorpion stings the turtle and they both drown with the Scorpion's deepest apology – "Sorry, but that's what I do."

This brings to mind the Walrus's lament in *Alice in Wonderland*, "We weep for you the Walrus cried, we deeply sympathize, as with sobs and tears he gobbled down those of largest size."

MW frequency has a cumulative effect. It may not bother you today but what about tomorrow which means it builds up inside and affects one according to the power of one's immune system to stand against the frequency. Prolonged exposure to microwave frequencies gravely compromises the immune system by affecting phagocytises, the immune response that removes dead and foreign cells. It seems phagocytes stop ingesting bacteria and other foreign bodies when exposed to prolonged MW frequency. Judging from photos of microwaved water crystals in Emoto's water books the effect appears immediate and powerful.

When I recently learned of the FCC proposal to eliminate land phone lines I was heartbroken. I knew if that occurred I would give up phone service. My decision is based on over 220 peer reviewed, published papers documenting the similarity between the effects of gamma waves and microwave radiation. The reports say the two are identically carcinogenic and genotoxic to the cellular roots of life. When one cannot afford possible ramifications, radical steps must be taken.

### Treatment

Looking at similarities between effects of radioactivity and microwave frequency radiation I thought it prudent to research a proven diet for exposure to radiation and found it in "How to Help Support the Body's Healing After Intense Radioactive or Radiation Exposure" by Bill Bodri found at **www.meditationexpert.com**. The report contains research and treatments used at the time of Hiroshima and Chernobyl. Seaweed saved the day for many victims.

Seaweeds contain sodium alginate which binds radioactive compounds including strontium, calcium, barium, cadmium and radium. Chernobyl victims were given 5 grams of Spirulina a day for 45 days. When tested by Institute of Radiation Medicine in Minsk the children showed enhanced immune systems & T cell counts and reduced radioactivity. Sounds real good – particularly when viewing Emoto's photos of microwaved water crystals.

There are other ways to combat the effect of MW frequency. I have been using Total Shield for over 5 years. It is a device 9 by 5 inches that contains several Tesla coils and claims to *"detect, interrupt and eliminate grid lines, geomagnetic, electromagnetic standing waves, E.L.F. and other harmful waves by broadcasting these disturbances through the Tesla Coil at a phase shift of 180 degrees. A second generator generates 7.83 earth resonant frequency. Total Shield blankets and protects a 20,000 square foot area."*

Cell phones and microwave technology are considered miracles of our time. So-called intelligent people claim life would be impossible without them. As with much superficial information–the opposite is true for a technology that totally disrupts family life, obliterates privacy, destroys the immune system and provides governments with a powerful system for controlling the masses.

I would love to drive the streets of America broadcasting over a loud speaker: *Wake up, wake-up, wake-up. You are no longer in control; your thoughts and feelings are being manipulated by the MW antennas distributed throughout every inch of your environment. Turn off your wireless devices, cell phones, and HD TV.*

## Appendix C

# The Big Stink

We are inundated with toxic artificial fragrances in the form of soaps, plug-ins, aerosols, room fresheners, fabric fresheners, perfumes, scented candles/oils and garbage bags. I opened a box of plastic garbage bags and became nauseas from a febreze-like odor. Gag!!!!!!!!!! Upon returning to the store I punched little holes in prospective boxes, large enough to catch a whiff of the inner contents before making another purchase.

Have you ever tried to remove the febreze odor from a fabric? If you frequent second-hand clothing shops and don't like that *fragrance*, beware - sniff out the garment before purchase, because the odor will not come out. It's there for all eternity. And if you are a traveler with sensitivities to artificial fragrances, it's a good idea to ask questions before checking into a motel.

Chemically sensitive city-folk have a hard time with the odor worn by thousands as a remnant of the laundry soap they use. When the stinkers make a quick exit from an elevator, subway, office etc. they leave the odor behind in a sea of ghastly fragrance.

It doesn't matter what fragrance-peddlers say regarding the safety of petrochemicals and exotic toxins; we know better. Artificial fragrances are composed of **untold** combinations of highly volatile petrochemical derivatives. The raw materials of perfumery are the solvents hexane and petroleum ether. According to a Natural Resource Defense Council sponsored test, 12 out of 14 air fresheners contain phthalates. These off-gassing chemicals are never listed as ingredients. They are claimed as proprietary secrets.

Perfumed garbage bags are created through a process that involves perfumed composites of ethylene and various copolymers such as vinyl acetate and ethyl acrylate which enable bags to retain fragrance for a year or more. Other types of perfumed objects are coated with polyurethane and essential oils to provide sustained release of aroma.

Procter and Gamble had to seek approval from the NYS Division of Solid and Hazardous Materials in order to register **Febreze Antimicrobial** because it contains Didecyl Dimethyl Ammonium Chloride. This product is used on fabrics to kill odor causing bacteria. The official letter from the Director of the Bureau of Pesticides Management states DDAC is a severe skin and eye irritant and goes on to say **"In the risk assessment conducted** by the U.S.EPA, post-application dermal exposures were determined to pose unacceptable risks." Yet – the product was given the O.K. for production. Wow. Imagine some of that stuff up against your skin for 10 hours.

Didecyl dimethyl ammonium chloride is listed as a *Pesticide Action Network (PAN) Bad Actor* meaning it is "acutely toxic". It is the most toxic ranking assigned by any organization. Read the info for yourself at Pan Pesticides Database under chemicals.

Keep artificial fragrances away from contact with children, animals and birds. The smaller the creature the greater are the possibilities for harm. Commercial cleaners should be avoided on floors where children, pets and yoga practitioners gather. You might want to try borax, vinegar and baking soda.

Most readers are familiar with air fresheners hanging from the rear view mirror of autos since the '60s. The chems emitted by the fresheners cling to dust particles which bond with chems in cigarette smoke, forming the dreaded phthalates.

Triclosan, a chemical used for antibacterial properties, is found in soaps, cosmetics, tooth paste, detergents and deodorants. It is registered as a pesticide by the EPA who claims it is a risk to humans, animals and the environment. "The chemical formulation and molecular structure of this compound are similar to some of the most toxic chemicals on earth, relating it to dioxins and PCBs."

Although over 70% of all liquid soap sold in the US contains triclosan, the 2005 Annals of Internal Medicine carried a study which found it did little to control symptoms of contagion; antibacterial soaps don't protect against viruses and most bacteria can be controlled with regular soap. Why is it so popular? We rely on commercials for our reality check and follow the dictates of corporate America.

Why use *little trees* when open windows will solve the problem. If fresh air doesn't work, try natural oils on pieces of felt – you can cut it to look like the tree or flower of your choice. Or hang a sachet of flowers and hide a sock full of baking soda under the seat.

I almost gave a toxic evergreen infusion as a gift. It looked great with a graceful diffusion system and pleasant aroma. There was no ingredient list – a dead give-a-way – so I called the company and discovered ½ of the content was a "cosmetic preservative". Just what one needs wafting about for the holidays.

Never has it been more important to know what you are putting into your personal environment. According to a 5/9/11 Time Magazine article – *Toxic Environment*, written by Alice Park only five chemicals have been regulated by the Toxic Substances Control Act (TSCA) of '76 in the past 30 years and the TSCA does not require any premarket testing of effects on human health.

I recall running away from atomizers on the move in NYC department stores. The moment one walked through the door, a rush of sales reps moved forward with awful smelling, artificial fragrances wafting the air. Often they became offended when one refused to be covered with their product.

Now days it's a pleasant surprise to find a store that does not have a strangely unpleasant odor throughout the entire floor. Perhaps a super sensitive nose is not equipped to withstand the onslaught of artificiality.

# Notes

- Heisenberg and Bohr discovered there's no such thing as solid reality. Objects in the material world are made up of subatomic particles that are constantly changing. Just as Castaneda described - bundles of energy are flying about, engaged in non-stop communication with the Field.

- Subatomic particles move out of invisibility when observed. As soon as a subatomic entity is measured it becomes real in the material world. This supports the long believed New Age philosophy that we create our individual realities. Experiments have been conducted using particle detectors which show that observed photons behave as solids.

- Research of the Field has revealed genes behave in the same manner as subatomic particles except that genes are modified by environment, life styles, diet and all we come in contact with. All of these gene-modifiers come from outside the body. I wonder how microwave frequency is modifying our genetic structure and the world as we know it.

- Research shows depression and fear weakens the immune system. MW frequency also weakens the immune system. Meditation and exercise will combat fear and depression. Removing MW devices from the home and living away from cell towers will allow the immune system to heal.

- Memory processes are emotion-driven, part of the unconscious and accessed via the right hemisphere of the brain.

- Within the Field, time doesn't exist; concepts of past and future are not relevant. Until a quantum event is observed, it exists only as a probability. The past and future live in the present moment. This supports the occurrence of remote viewing and other psychic events.

- The memory of events occurring in a place, leaves a permanent record which can be accessed long after the events.

- The Quantum world is a single, gigantic field of energy that is slowed down, and only shows tendencies to exist; it is a product of individual consciousness and implies we are the Whole, not parts of a whole as LB deductive reasoning seems to suggest. Wouldn't it be wonderful to introduce these concepts as a game of wonder in primary school grades? Perhaps it would generate students interested in pursuing science.

- HAARP stands for High Frequency Active Auroral Research Program. According to Wikipedia the Ionospheric Research Instrument (IRI) is a high power radio frequency transmitter operating in the high MW frequency band and used to excite the upper portion of the atmosphere. HAARP conspiracy theory says it is used to heat up regions on the planet to direct hurricanes and create tsunamis and earthquakes. It would be difficult to determine who is doing what since the U.S., Russia, France, Australia, Iran, Peru, Puerto Rico, Norway, Sweden and Japan have gigantic HAARP installations with "antenna farms" capable of pulsing *weather war frequencies* across the planet. According to Google there are HAARP farms all over America creating rings of frequency viewable on the internet.
- Eileen and Peter Caddy and Dorothy Maclean were disciplined meditators before coming to live at the Findhorn Caravan where they continued meditation practices which offered guidance for the garden initially started out of necessity.

The garden, on barren, sandy, windswept coastal Scotland, began to flourish when meditation led them to communicate with the forces of nature such as Pan, devas and elemental beings of the plant world. These "overlighting forces" of the "formless energy field" led them to grow enormous plants, dozens of species of flowers and fruits and the world famous 40 pound cabbages.

In *The Findhorn Garden* they write of Pan's "light body" and tell of a first encounter with him. "The moment he (Pan) stepped into me the woods became alive with myriad beings – elementals, nymphs, dryads, fauns, elves, gnomes, fairies and so on, far too numerous to catalogue."

It is an amazing, inspiring story of a garden that continues to thrive today. There is much that confirms the material found in Napoleon's Bathtub. It is a must read for gardeners working in difficult environmental conditions.

# Random Thoughts

Early education in America must change. RB modes need to be encouraged in order to achieve Bimodal consciousness. Otherwise children grades 1 – 12 will continue to lose interest and eventually drop out. If the student is not interested in what is going on they will not learn. A seed of emotional content must be embedded in all concepts, ideas, skills and philosophies presented.

ⓞⓞⓞⓞⓞ

Females in K – 3rd grade excel in LB processing. Such is not the case with little boys who start school with all the delightful abilities bestowed by RB dominance. Their sports abilities are outstanding while girls often sit on the sideline. Initially, boys are at a disadvantage with LB strategies such as reading and math and should be allowed to start school a year later. This is accepted information that is not being acted upon. Like many arenas, from politics to medicine, answers are available but action is not forthcoming.

Protect your male child from being labeled and medicated. Hold back on Kindergarten and monitor the 1st grade process by staying in weekly contact with the teacher. Or send your male children to a Waldorf or Montessori school.

ⓞⓞⓞⓞⓞⓞⓞⓞ

We are living histories of our current and past lives. Our health is a testament to our beliefs, actions, and emotional life. Not only do we create ourselves, we create the world around us. Do what one must to avoid depression, negativity, fear and harmful environmental conditions.

ⓞⓞⓞⓞⓞⓞⓞ

Chief Seattle had a clear image of the Field when he said "All things are connected like the blood which unites one family. Whatever befalls the earth befalls the sons of earth. Man did not weave the web of life, he is merely a strand of it. Whatever he does to the web, he does to himself."

ⓞⓞⓞⓞⓞⓞ

Love necessitates care; without care there is no love. When you don't love yourself there is no ability to love others. These are excellent signs of what is really going on in relationships.

ⓞⓞⓞⓞⓞⓞ

Martial arts and meditation are excellent disciplines for young children.

# Bibliography

Atwater, P.M.H. *Future Memory*. Moment Point Press, 2002.

Batmanghelidj, F. MD. *Your Body's Many Cries for Water*. Global Health Solutions, Inc. 1997.

Bartholomew, Sandy. *Yoga for Your Brain*. Design Originals, 2011.

Begich, Nick. *Angles Don't Play This HAARP*. Earthpulse Press, 1995.

Bentov, Itzhak. *Stalking the Wild Pendulum*. E.P. Dutton, 1977.

Bird, Christopher. *The Divining Hand*. Whitford Press, 1993.

Bohm, David. *Wholeness and the Implicate Order*. Routledge & Kegan Paul, 1980.

Brakeslee, Thomas R. *The Right Brain*. Anchor Press/Doubleday, 1980.

Brennan, Barbara. *Hands of Light*. Bantam Books, 1987.

Campbell, Colin & Thomas. *The China Study*. Benbella Books, 2006.

Caputo, Robert. *Tang Soo Tao – The Living Buddha in Martial Virtue*. Coleman's Printing Pty. Ltd, 1981.

Carlo, Dr. George & Schram, Martin. *Cell Phones*. Carroll & Graf Publishers, 2001.

Castaneda, Carlos. *A Separate Reality*. Washington Square Press, 1971.

Cohen MD, Gene D. *The Creative Age*. Quill/Harper Collins, 2000.

David-Neel, Alexandra & Lama Yongden. *The Secret Oral Teachings in Tibetan Buddhist Sects*. City Lights Books, 1967.

Dimond, Stuart J. & Beaumont, J. Graham. *Hemisphere Function in the Human Brain*. John Wiley & Sons, 1974.

Durckheim, Karlfried Graf Von. Hara, *The Vital Centre of Man*. Mandala Books, 1977.

Edwards, Betty. *Drawing on the Right Side of the Brain*. Jeremy P. Tarcher Inc, 1989.

Emoto, Masaru. *The Hidden Messages in Water*. Atria Books, 2001.

Findhorn Community. *The Findhorn Garden*. Harper Colophon Books, 1975.

Frantzis, Bruce Kumar. *The Power of Internal Martial Arts*. North Atlantic Books, 1998.

Gedgaudas, Nora T. *Primal Body, Primal Mind*. Healing Arts Press, 2011.

Gribbin, John. *In Search of Schrodinger's Cat*. Bantam Books, 1984.

Haich, Elizabeth. *Initiation*. Seed Center, 1974.

Hanh, Thich Nhat. *No death, No Fear*. Riverhead Books/Penguin Putnam, 2002.

Hyams, Joe. *Zen in the Martial Arts*. J.P. Tarcher Inc, 1979.

Inayat-Khan, Pir Vilayat. *Toward the One*. Harper Colophon Books, 1974.

James, John PhD. *The Great Field*. Elite Books, 2007.

Leadbeater, W. C. *The Chakras*. The Theosophical Publishing House, 1972.

Lee, Bruce. *Tao of Jeet Dune Do*. Ohara Publications, 1975.

Lipton, Bruce H. *The Biology of Belief*. Hay House Inc, 2005.

Masunaga, Shizuto with Wataru Ohashi. *Zen Shiatsu*. Japan Publications, 1977.

McTaggart, Lynne. *The Field*. Quill/Harper Collins Publishers, 2002.

Motoyama, Hiroshi. *Theories of the Chakras: Bridge to Higher Consciousness*. Theosophical Publishing House, 1981.

Mundy, Talbot. *Om, The Secret of Abhor Valley*. Crown Publishers, 1924.

Ohashi, Wataru. *Do It Yourself Shiatsu*. E.P. Dutton, 1976.

Ouspensky, P.D. *In Search of the Miraculous*. Harcourt Brace Jovanovich, 1949.

Pearce, Joseph Chilton. *Crack in the Cosmic Egg*. Washington Square Press; 1971.

Payne, Peter. *Martial Arts – The Spiritual Dimension*. Crossroad, 1981.

Rees, Camilla & Magda Havas. *Public Health SOS: The Shadow Side of the Wireless Revolution*. Wide Angle Health, 2009.

Renard, Gary R. *The Disappearance of the Universe*. Fearless Books, 2003.

Schapiro, Mark. *Exposed*. Chelsea Green Publishing, 2007.

Segalowitz, Sid J. *Two Sides of the Brain*. Prentice Hall Inc, 1983.

Smith, Jeffrey M. *Seeds of Deception*. Yes Books, 2003.

Talbot, Michael. *The Holographic Universe*. Harper Perennial, 1992.

Targ, Russell & Harold E. Puthoff. *Mind Reach*. Delacorte Press, 1977.

Tart, Charles T. *Open Mind, Discriminating Mind*. Harper & Row, 1989.

Tipler, Frank J. *The Physics of Immortality*. Anchor Books/Doubleday, 1994.

Tolstoy, Alexandra. *Tolstoy, A life of My Father*. Harper & Brothers, 1953.

Vivekananda, Swami. *Raja Yoga*. Ramakrishna-Vivekananda Center, 1956.

Wolf, Fred Allan. *Parallel Universes*. Simon and Schuster, 1988.

**Reports**

"Bioeffects of Non-lethal Weapons". U.S. Army National Ground Intelligence Center Study, 1998.

Dubey, R.BB & M. Hanmandlu & S.K. Gupta. "Risk of Brain Tumors from Wireless Phone Use". Journal of Computer Assisted Tomography, Nov/Dec, 2010.

www.ingramcontent.com/pod-product-compliance
Lightning Source LLC
Chambersburg PA
CBHW052133270326
41930CB00012B/2872